BLU ROOM®

Experience the future
Building bridges with light, frequency, and sound

Irmgard Maria Gräf

For more information about the Blu Room contact: Blu Room Enterprises, LLC, P.O. Box 5895, Lacey, WA 98509, USA. www.bluroom.com

ISBN-13: 978-1547129157
ISBN-10: 1547129158

Exceptional thinkers, scientists and visionaries inspired this book. Thanks to their discoveries, explorations, critical research, genius expertise and writings, the book evolved into this volume. This book presents my best and most serious attempt to comprehensively present available evidence in a coherent, explanatory reference system. Not everything has to be proven to experience it.

The book unfolds step by step. Each topic opens up a broader range of knowledge, an immersing into exciting dimensions. The book stimulates thought and calls on new paradigms to be questioned and fascinating worlds to be experienced.

Let us explore the world of light, frequencies and sound, and prepare to experience the medicine of the future close up!

CONTENTS

Pulsating Life

Light is a fascinating mystery which is present everywhere. It is of fundamental importance to all life on our planet. Light affects not only the quality of food, but also our physical, mental and spiritual health. In unimaginable ways, it controls all the energy fields of our organisms.

Without light there is no life. Plants use the power of sunlight to create a living entity out of a single seed with the help of water, carbon dioxide, mineral salts and trace elements.

Each plant, and of course every animal, is a unity. Where does this order come from? Who is the programmer of this process? It may only be sunlight. Living systems depend on taking order or signal energy from their environment to establish and promote their congenital order. Light has profound effects on all organisms.

The physics of elementary particles, the physics of the cosmos, and the biology of life itself – all connect.

The goal of this book is to encourage you to explore, appreciate and bolster the remarkable richness of life itself and our world.

Take a breathtaking journey into little known worlds.

Chapter One

Biophotons - The Light in our Cells

A brilliantly simple experiment

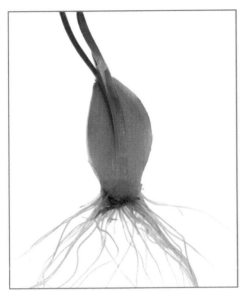

In the 1920s, the Russian research couple Lydia and Alexander Gurwitsch led a brilliantly simple experiment. Gurwitsch had already done extended research on embryology. He knew that in the process of embryonic development, the number of cells increases as they divide. In this unique "onion" experiment Gurwitsch and his scientist wife questioned which factors cause cell reproduction. Cells of onion roots were known to divide rapidly yet still retain the circular cross-section. This is crucial for the onion form. Gurwitsch assumed that the cells emit radiation during cell division and thus influence the cell division of the other cells.

They positioned an onion root so that the tip of this first onion root pointed to the side of another onion root. They did not touch each other. After a while Gurwitsch investigated these two onion roots under a microscope and saw "at exactly the point of near-contact, there was a significant increase of cell divisions (mitosis) compared to the opposite side." The effect disappeared when a thin piece of window glass or other material was placed between the two roots. This material is opaque to ultraviolet light. The "mitogenetic effect" reappeared when the ordinary glass was replaced with quartz glass, which is transparent for ultraviolet light. (1) Gurwitsch kept repeating this experiment to finally to prove that the force behind this mitogenetic effect was a very weak ultraviolet radiation emanating from the tip of the first onion root. He called this "mitogenetic radiation" (1) Dr. Alexander Gurwitsch published the results 1923. (2)

Two identical cells through mitosis

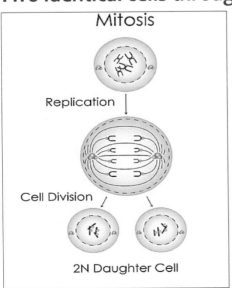

Mitosis

Replication

Cell Division

2N Daughter Cell

Life is based on the ability of cells to reproduce, or make copies of themselves. This is done by a process called cell-division. One cell divides into two. This is not a random process. The cell prepares for this division by initially making a copy of the innate DNA. Each new cell shall receive this complete set of chromosomes. The result is the transformation of one cell into two identical daughter cells. The Polish histologist Waclaw Mayzel was the first to describe 1875 this process. He called it "mitosis." Mitosis plays an important role for all living beings. In a human body ten million cells die per second and ten million new cells are built anew. A correct mitosis is crucial.

In 1944 the quantum physicist, Erwin Schrödinger, introduced the idea of the human being a carrier, transmitter and storage of information in his book *What is life?* (3) .Thus he spurred the thoughts of Prof. Dr. Fritz-Albert Popp. Schrödinger wrote, "We observed from higher animals, when they eat foods, they achieve symmetry in their systems." He also explains: "Plants have the strongest stock of sunlight." From this storage we humans receive energy and signals at a cellular level. Popp developed this idea further and introduced this concept of information in molecular biology. In 1975 he succeeded in the experimental proof of biophotons.

Countless researchers from all over the world keep confirming the light emission of all cells in all living things. It is an extremely weak light, which increases during cell division, damage or near death. As soon as the cell is dead, the weak light emission is gone. (3)

Secret life inside

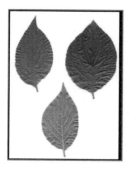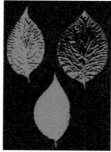

Dan Eden, author of *Is DNA the next internet*, talks about the first documentations at the International Institute of Biophysics:

"Dr. Popp opens a big wooden box. He places a fresh cutting from a plant and a wooden match in a plastic container inside this dark box and closes the light proof door. He then activates the photomultiplier. An image appears on a computer screen. The match stick is black while the green, glowing silhouette of the leaves is clearly visible." (4)

On the left: leaves in daylight.
On the right: the biophoton emission of the same leaves shown by a photomultiplier.

Surely, if the leaves could emit a light in the photomultiplier, then all living beings would do the same. Dr. Popp is excited: "We now know that man is essentially a being of light." (4)

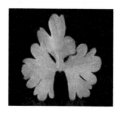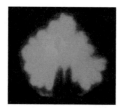

The parsley transforms into a gentle luminous being under the photomultiplier.

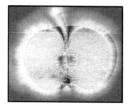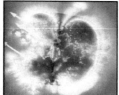

The biophoton field reflects the healthy and a spoiled apple.
Source: International Institute of Biophysics, Neuss, Germany

All living cells of plants, animals and human beings emit biophotons. Popp expanded the Gurwitsch discovery and revealed that DNA was at the origin of biophotons and measured their coherence. He developed a biophoton theory to explain their possible biological role and the ways in which they may control biochemical processes, growth, differentiation etc. Biophotons cannot be seen by the naked eye but they can be measured by special equipment. German researchers developed such a device. It is called a photomultiplier.

Biophotons versus photons

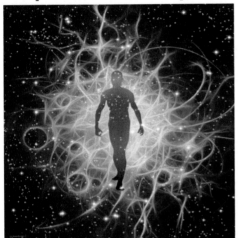

The idea of the photon originates from Albert Einstein's work on the photoelectric effect in 1905. In 1926, the American physical chemist, Gilbert Lewis, established the physical reality of photons.

Photons are elementary particles of light. The photon has zero rest mass and is always moving at the speed of light. Biophotons are photons as well. Their only peculiarity is that they derive from biological systems. They differ from normal photons, because they have the property of being measurable when examining living systems. Popp proved that every living substance emits a dim light with wavelengths between 200 and 800 nanometers, especially in a tight range of UVB radiation.

In quantum electrodynamics the photon is a mediator of the electromagnetic interaction in the gauge bosons.

Biophotons are tiny light particles, which operate in all living organisms as information carriers. They control about one trillion metabolic processes per second. Biophotons are the light in the cells of all living things; they are alive, vibrant and highly structured coherent light with the ability of interference and the superposition of waves, allowing information to be transferred. Every living organism must be a light system. Every living organism, even the grass, the walnut, the swallow, the ant, the earthworm, the dog, the neighbor, the postman and the crying boy are organisms filled with radiant cells.

We walk within an obvious and yet invisible light field, with different light beings and their thoughts. (5)

Biophotons are quanta of ultra-weak cell radiation. Their intensity is approximately 10^{18} times weaker than ordinary daylight. Their visibility is 1,000 times lower than the sensitivity of our naked eye. The intensity corresponds to the brightness of a candle, which is viewed from 20 km away. While not visible to us, these particles of light are part of the visible electromagnetic spectrum (380-780 nm) and are detectable via sophisticated modern instruments. (6) "However," says Popp "regardless of their delicacy biophotons possess a tremendous consistency and thus a high degree of order." It is precisely this quality that brings equilibrium to the surrounding system. This makes it the most important key factor to understanding the complete biochemistry, indeed the origin of life. (7)

Resonance between waves and particles

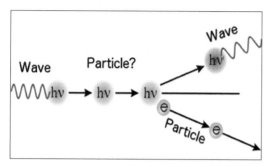

Wave–particle duality is the concept that every elementary particle or quantum entity may behave either as a wave or as a particle, depending on the circumstances. John Gribbin, the author of the encyclopedia *Q is for Quantum* writes: "a particle is usually regarded as having a precise location in space, but a wave is intrinsically a spread-out thing, and the uncertainty in the position of, say, an electron can be linked to its wave nature." (8)

Quantum physics speak of the wave-particle duality of light. The simultaneity of both counterparts in nature is observed as a true coherent state. (9) For Prof. Popp "Biophotons are created by resonance between waves and particles. They are the intermediary and the indicator of a dynamic equilibrium or the product of a bipolar coherent state between the waves and particles." (7)

In 1951 Albert Einstein remarked, in a letter to his old friend Michelangelo Besso: 'All these fifty years of conscious brooding have brought me no nearer to the answer to the question "what are light quanta?" Nowadays every Tom, Dick and Harry thinks he knows it, but he is mistaken.' According to John Gribbin this still holds true as we approach the end of the 20th century, nearly 100 years after Einstein started brooding about light. (8)

Many years have passed and researchers are stepping further ahead into the unknown, unravelling unexpected phenomena.

Coherent light is the principle of order

Coherent light waves are light waves of the same wavelength and the same phase. According to the ideas of the coherence theory of biophotons, there is a coherent light composite between the DNA

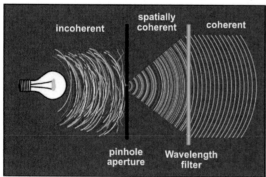

and all other cell components in the cell. Its main role is attributed to this light and controls of the biochemical-material processes. The scientists at the International Institute of Biophysics in Neuss assumed that this is "due to the fact that all biochemical processes are the result of the excitation of photons and the coherence of light. Such a light compound is an ideal medium for the transmission of information." (5)

Source: www.ryerson.ca

Dance between chaos and order

The high degree of order is referred to in physics as coherence. Popp proved that biophotons are characterized by an extremely high degree of order and structure. Living systems like living cells and living beings are not always in a high-coherent state, but rather "oscillate at the so-called laser threshold between order and disorder. Thus they can jump back and forth between degrees of order and, in the extreme case, by exchanging a single photon they can jump between order and disorder." (10)

The coherence of a system's biophoton field describes its vitality and its energy state. "Coherent states or the state of the biophoton field are an indicator of the extent to which a system resonates in harmony with its environment. It can record new potential information, wave aspects and can then harmonize, shape-build or system-sustain with the current information, the particle aspect."(5)

The processes of morphogenesis, growth, differentiation and regeneration are also demonstrated by the structuring and regulating activity of the coherent biophoton field. The neurophysiologist Karl Pribram and his team assume that "the holographic biophoton field of the brain and the nervous system, and maybe even that of the whole organism, may also be a basis of memory and other phenomena of consciousness." (11) The consciousness-like coherent properties of the biophoton field – "are closely related to the properties of the physical vacuum and indicate the biophoton field's possible role as an interface to the non-physical realms of mind, psyche and consciousness." (12)

The research results of Rupert Sheldrake show an evident morphogenetic field. Prof Dr. Popp said in an interview in Munich in 1999, "I am more and more inclined to give even Sheldrake's considerations more contemplation for the following reason: In quantum theory non-electromagnetic interactions supported by Sheldrake are of great importance." (13)

Dr. Peter Garjajev assumes that this kind of communication does not merely occur within individual cells or between two individual cells. Organisms use this "light" to communicate with other organisms. (14)

There is much evidence that the biophoton radiation of living cells not only covers more than just the range of visible light. It acts like a radio transmitter for cells. The signals in the organisms of plants, animals and humans control biological processes with far greater speed and efficiency than via biochemical channels. A 2010 study states, "cell to cell communication by biophotons has been demonstrated in plants, bacteria, animal neutrophil granulocytes and kidney cells." Researchers found that "different spectral light stimulation (infrared, red, yellow, blue, green and white) at one end of the spinal sensory or motor nerve roots resulted in a significant increase in the biophotonic activity at the other end." (15)

Science revealed that photons are essential to the basic health and function of DNA and are apparently used to send and receive information throughout the body. Each DNA molecule is believed to store up to 1,000 photons similar to that of a tiny fiber-optic cable. In 2017, Lance

Shuttler published new scientific experiments to validate that "DNA begins as a Quantum Wave and not as a Molecule." He writes, "The photons shoot back and forth at the speed of light inside the molecule and are stored until they needed." (16)

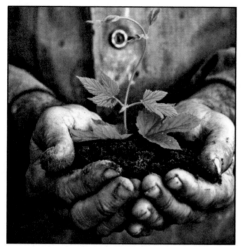

The American scientist, Lubert Stryer, discovered a biophoton radiation in the infrared range in his investigations of mitochondrial metabolism, this biophoton was released by electrons from nutrients. He recognized "that this infrared radiation "charged" the ATP molecules." (17)

When nutrients decay, they release not only heat, but also electromagnetic energy. At the same time, this infrared biophoton radiation of the cell is also available as a direct energy source. In contrast to heat, biophoton radiation in the infrared range is directly accessible energy for movement, synapse transmission of the neurons and any kind of cellular activity. (18) The ability of our mitochondria to produce a powerful biophoton field with little effort and no toxic burden is the key to our health and evolution.

Popp's biophoton theory leads to many startling insights into our life processes and may well provide one of the major elements for new inventions and applications in the field of medicine and technology.

The discovery of biophoton emissions also lends scientific support to some unconventional methods of healing based on concepts of homeostasis, a self-regulation of the organism. Various somatic therapies, homeopathy and acupuncture depend on the presence of coherent and structured light. The "chi" energy flowing in our energy channels may be related to the node lines of the organism's biophoton field. The "prana" of Indian Yoga physiology may be a similar regulating energy force that has a basis in weak, coherent electromagnetic biofields. (19)

It was only logical...

Excerpt of an interview with Prof. Dr. Fritz A. Popp 1999
Pioneer of light and frequency

Q. How did you get the idea that cells emit light and that this light is used for communication, i.e. the exchange of information in the body's processes? This breaks a scientific taboo, by trusting that light exchanges intelligent information and thus brings a new meaning to the processes of life! (20)

Dr. Popp: "It was only logical! Every second a person loses 10^7 cells or in other words: when I say 21, 22, ten million cells have died! Every 10^7 seconds a signal must be transmitted to the neighboring cells, which transmit-the message of the cell loss! This so-called cell loss rate is valid for all biological systems, i.e. for all living beings. However, the entire organism must constantly be aware of these

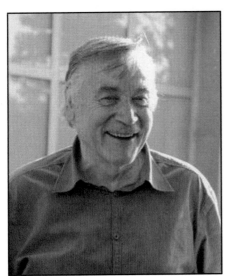

cell losses, otherwise tumors will arise or not enough cells will be reproduced. The integrity of the body depends on this. But how can this immense information exchange of billions of dead cells per day take place anyway? On what basis can you organize such a thing? Electrochemical processes would not be capable of handling this jumble of errands in such short intervals. Erwin Schrödinger wondered at that time, why biology made no mistakes despite the immense number of reactions that take place at any given moment. With this amount, the operations would actually be completely chaotic." (13)

Source: www.naturscheck.de

The exciting field of research of the physicist Prof. Dr. Popp is nothing less than life itself. His findings provide scientists with a new view of the processes in the human body, the principle of our life and other lifeforms in outer dimensions. Communication primarily takes place through light.

"There are about 100,000 chemical reactions happening in every cell each second. The chemical reaction can only happen if the reacting molecule is excited by a photon. Once the photon has enkindled a reaction it returns to the field and is available for more reactions. We are swimming in an ocean of light." Prof. Dr. Fritz-Albert Popp is convinced. (18)

Man is a light eater

"Man," says physicist Popp "is not a meat eater or a vegetarian. It is a light mammal - Incredible as some may think: There is light in our cells. It pulsates and acts in a way very much alive, as if it breathes like waving leaves in the wind."

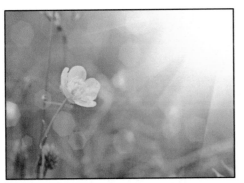

When we eat, light energy passes through our organism. Light controls all biochemical processes in connection with the body's own information. The higher the light storage capability of the food, the higher is the contribution of cellular order.

All animals and people feed directly or indirectly from plants. So we eat indirect sunlight. Sunlight is hence more or less the cell code of biological light - the key of life. Light improves our quality of life. The Nobel laureate David Bohm and Albert Szent-Gyorgyi were convinced decades ago: "All energy that we ingest into our bodies comes from the sun, either directly or indirectly through food". (21)

Dr. Johanna Budwig, world's leading authority on fatty acids speaks of a resonance system: "The electrons in food act as a resonance system for solar energy. The vital photons play the part of life elements. They are adjusted according to the quantum resonance with the electrons in seed oils on the wavelength of the solar energy. This interaction dominates all life functions."(22)

What do we actually eat?

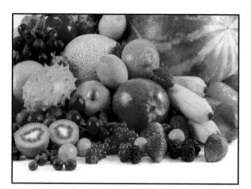

Nobel laureate and physicist Erwin Schrödinger recognized that order in the human body is established through living food. If we eat fresh and energetic food, we improve the harmony in our body.

The higher the light content and thus the vital information in the food, the more suitable it is to regulate the system of the cells in the body. "With regard to food, the light level is more important than the content composition of nutrients such as carbohydrates, protein, vitamins and minerals. Inferior foods lead to degeneration of cell communication in our organism." (23)

Light storage capacity

The light storage capacity of food is the decisive criterion for its quality. Quality of food is the degree of regulatory power that it provides to a consumer. The higher the light storage capacity of the food as a whole is, the better the integration of light into the living organism. The better the light storage order is, the higher is the biological quality.

Prof. Popp and his team in Germany built a special photomultiplier tube instrument to measure biophotonic emission. The apple, as an example, is irradiated in a light-tight chamber with a defined light quantity and quality. The photomultiplier is then used to measure how much light is emitted, and how stable the light storage capacity of the food is.

The Redox potential

The physical grade measuring system of high biophoton activity is referred to as redox potential. As early as 1968 Werner Kollath wrote in his book *Regulators of Life - the knowledge of the redox systems,* "The properties of the food depend on how well they can emit electrons and thus render free radicals harmless. The lower the millivolt value of the food, the greater its ability to deliver electrons to other compounds and therefore to trap more free radicals."(6)

Every second 10 million cells die in our bodies. This loss must be replaced. This means our body will constantly create new life out of the ingredients available. If our organism permanently receives food weak in light and failing biophotons, the cell- and life-regeneration lack the conditions for vitality and health. The aging process is accelerated and the risk of disease increases.

Chlorophyll is a mediator between light and food

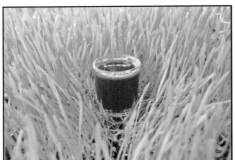

Plants absorb the light of the sun, the water of the earth, and the carbon dioxide from the air. They build their own carbohydrates in form of sugar or starch. Chlorophyll is the molecule that absorbs sunlight and uses its energy to synthesize carbohydrates from CO_2 and water. This process is known as photosynthesis. Chlorophyll is the green part in leaves.

Since animals and humans secure their food supply by eating plants, photosynthesis can be seen as a life-sustaining element.

The light value of our food

- Organic fruits and vegetables have a higher biophoton radiation than conventionally grown plants.
- Fresh and especially wild herbs carry a wealth of biophotons and at the same time healing agents.
- Spices (such as aniseed, cinnamon, cocoa, carob, cardamom, galangal, turmeric and ginger) stimulate circulation and happiness. They stimulate not only the taste buds, but also activate the metabolism of biophotons.
- Animal products are important suppliers of nutrients especially when grown appropriate to their species.

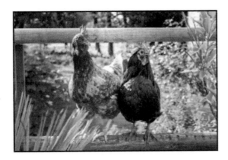

Scientists at the International Institute of Biophysics (IIB) have ascertained in many experiments, that significant differentiators are evident in the biophoton radiation of chicken eggs in free-range and from battery hens. (24). The results indicated that organic eggs showed higher emissions of biophotons with a slower decline, higher albumen height, paler yolk color, and higher content of omega-3 fatty acids in yolks. (25)

- Food from industrial production, food stored in the refrigerator or the freezer for a long time or food cooked in the microwave, has low or no biophoton concentration. Flavor enhancers and other chemical substances destroy downright light.
- Hydroponics and genetically modified foods with artificially generated properties have a low value of biophotons.
- Greenhouse plants under artificial lighting or harvested unripe have a weak biophoton capacity.
- Long transports diminish biophotons.

Professor Popp is convinced: "Everything heated, pasteurized, cooked, baked, canned, cooked in the microwave, frozen or otherwise denatured, is in a sense unlighted and thus dead."

Health therefore corresponds to a state of perfect communication. Illness indicates the breakdown of the light providing system and therefore disorder in cell-to-cell-communication. We get sick when our cells lose their synchronicity, their coherence.

The vital building blocks

Proteins - Amino Acids
Carriers of life
Proteins are essential for physical life. These vital amino acids are the building blocks of cells. They should be eaten exclusively in a natural, well digestible form. Protein is constantly required for all aspects of the metabolic processes.

The body needs protein for
- ✓ the immune system,
- ✓ the cell structure - muscles, bones, skin, hair, etc.,
- ✓ the structure of enzymes and hormones,
- ✓ the transmission of nerve impulses,
- ✓ the transport of oxygen and fats,
- ✓ the structure of collagen, antibodies, clotting factors, etc.

For proper protein metabolism, it is necessary that all the amino acids are in the right proportion to each other. If an amino acid is missing, the whole recovery process becomes disarrayed.

Fat and Fatty Acids
Sun for the brain
Fat or fatty acids are essential in a healthy diet. They are an important source of energy for the human organism. Fats are essential for the stability and flexibility of the body, especially in the cell membrane

The body needs living fat and fatty acids
- ✓ They are vital for the brain to receive pulses to store and retransmit properly and retrieve information and nutrients.
- ✓ They are important building factors for all cell membranes keeping them flexible and adaptable to communication.
- ✓ They are essential factors for development of oxygen and constant cellular respiration.
- ✓ They store and process sunlight, photon energy.
- ✓ They bind the fat soluble vitamins A, D, E and K.
- ✓ They store highly concentrated energy.
- ✓ They are essential for the function of hormones and enzymes.
- ✓ They reduce fluctuations in blood sugar levels.
- ✓ They protect organs and regulate body temperature.

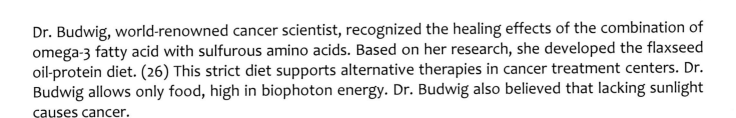

Dr. Budwig, world-renowned cancer scientist, recognized the healing effects of the combination of omega-3 fatty acid with sulfurous amino acids. Based on her research, she developed the flaxseed oil-protein diet. (26) This strict diet supports alternative therapies in cancer treatment centers. Dr. Budwig allows only food, high in biophoton energy. Dr. Budwig also believed that lacking sunlight causes cancer.

Carbohydrates
Fuel for life actions and a guarantee for cell to cell communication
Carbohydrates are crucial for energy, building blocks and serve as action mediators.

The body needs living carbohydrates
- ✓ They build fast and easily storable energy.
- ✓ They metabolize in glucose. The brain cells, erythrocytes and red blood cells depend on carbohydrates. They meet their energy needs exclusively from glucose.
- ✓ They are important for support functions. Complex carbohydrates are constituents of bones, tendons and connective tissue.
- ✓ They are an important energy reserve. Carbohydrates are stored as glycogen in the liver and in the muscles.
- ✓ Carbohydrates are constituents of blood group substances and anticoagulant substances.
- ✓ They regulate water and electrolyte balance.
- ✓ They have a protein-saving function.
- ✓ They are essential for active cell to cell communication.

Vitamins, enzymes and trace elements hold key functions in the organism.

Food is light. Light is ultimately the result of energy and information.

Metabolism
Metabolism is a term that is used to describe all chemical reactions involved in maintaining the living state of the cells and the organism. The metabolism of substances is dependent on the accompanying information and the light coherence. Nutrition is the key to metabolism. Metabolism is as individual and unique as human DNA.

The DNA as light storage and light source
According to the biophoton theory developed on the base of these discoveries, the biophoton light is stored in the cells of the organism - more precisely, in the DNA molecules of their nuclei. A dynamic web of light constantly released and absorbed by the DNA connects cell organelles, cells, tissues, and organs within the body. It serves as the organism's main communication network and as the principal regulating instance for all life processes. The importance of this discovery has been confirmed by scientists such as Herbert Froehlich (27) and Nobel laureate, Ilya Prigogine. (28)

The Creating Principle

Chapter Two

DNA – the Creating Principle

The discovery of the DNA

It begins in the 1800s…

In 1842, Karl Wilhelm von Nägeli discovered subcellular structures that would later became known as chromosomes. He had observed a network of string like bodies.

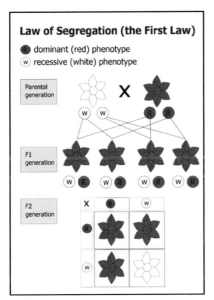

Law of Segregation (the First Law)
- ® dominant (red) phenotype
- ⓦ recessive (white) phenotype

Parental generation

F1 generation

F2 generation

In 1866 Gregor Mendel, the "Father of Genetics," published his results of his research on the inheritance of "factors" in pea plants. As a result, a flood of research began to try to prove or invalidate his theories. Are physical characteristics inherited from one generation to the next? (29)

In 1869 Swiss physiological chemist, Friedrich Miescher, identified what he called "nuclein" inside the nuclei of human white blood cells. The term "nuclein" was later changed to "nucleic acid" and eventually to "deoxyribonucleic acid," or "DNA." (30)

In 1879 Walther Flemming, an anatomist from Germany, discovered a fibrous structure within the nucleus of cells. He named this structure 'chromatin.' He had actually discovered chromosomes. By observing this chromatin, Flemming accurately figured out how chromosomes separate during cell division, also known as mitosis. (31)

In 1881 Albrecht Kossel, a German biochemist, identified nuclein as a nucleic acid and coined its present chemical name, deoxyribonucleic acid (DNA). He also isolated the five nucleotide bases. These are the building blocks of DNA and RNA: adenine (A), cytosine (C), guanine (G), thymine (T) and uracil (U). For his work he received the Nobel Prize in Physiology or Medicine in 1910. (29)

In 1928 Frederick Griffith, a scientist, worked on a theory that "DNA was the molecule of inheritance." Griffith's experiment involved mice and two types of pneumonia – one was virulent and the other non-virulent. He discovered the transfer of traits in these two forms of Pneumococcus. (29)

In 1929 Russian biochemist, Phoebus Levene, determined the order of the three major components of a single nucleotide (phosphate-sugar-base), the carbohydrate component of RNA (ribose), the carbohydrate component of DNA (deoxyribose). He also identified the way RNA and DNA molecules are put together. (29)

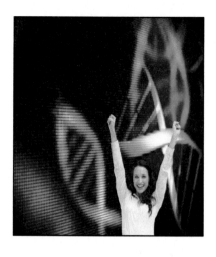

In 1940 an Austrian scientist, Erwin Chargaff, discovered the arrangement of the amounts of the four bases: adenine, guanine, cytosine, and thymine. This revelation later became Chargaff's Rule. (32) In May 1952, Chargaff met Watson and Crick informally in Cambridge, UK, and gave them the important ratio 1:1.

In his autobiography, Chargaff writes, "When I began to realize how unique the regularities were that we had discovered, I tried, of course, to understand what it all meant, but did not get very far. I attempted to build molecular models of the nucleotides... but I ran out of atoms and even more of patience." (33)

In 1951 two researchers, Rosalind Franklin and Maurice Wilkins, were successful in obtaining an x-ray pattern of a crystal of the DNA molecule. The pattern appeared to contain rungs, like those on a ladder between two strands that were side by side. Rosalind Franklin contributed to the discovery of the molecular structure of DNA.

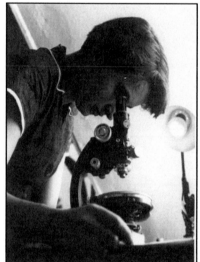

In 1953 Watson and Crick combined the known knowledge and proposed the Double Helix in the magazine *Nature*.

The English researchers Rosalind Franklin and Maurice Wilkins set the groundwork for Watson and Crick's derivation of the three-dimensional, double-helical model for the structure of DNA. Watson and Crick's discovery was also made possible by recent advances in model building, or the assembly of possible three-dimensional structures based on known molecular distances and bond angles. Watson and Crick shared Nobel Prize in Physiology or Medicine. (34)

Source: Profiles in Science Rosalind Franklin

In 1984 DNA profiling was developed a few years later by English geneticist Alec Jeffreys of the University of Leicester, and was used primarily to convict Colin Pitchfork in 1988 in the Enderby murders case in Leicestershire, England. Thus began the journey of DNA research. (35)

In 2008 Dr. Sergey Leikin caught micro gravitational effects generated by DNA in action. David Wilcock describes an experiment done by Leikin in his recent book *The Synchronicity Key*, "He put different types of DNA in regular salt water and marked each type with a different fluorescent color and the DNA molecules were then scattered throughout the water. Matching DNA molecules were then found pairing together. After a short time, entire clusters of the same colored DNA molecules had formed. Thus, it appears that DNA generates a micro gravitational effect that attracts and captures light." (36)

In **2011** Nobel Prize winner, Dr. Luc Montagnier, demonstrated that DNA can be built spontaneously merely out of hydrogen and oxygen. In his book *Synchronicity Key* Wilcox talks about this breathtaking discovery. "Montagnier started out with a hermetically sealed tube of pure sterilized water and then placed another sealed tube next to it. He had placed a small amount of DNA floating in water in the latter tube. Montagnier then electrified both tubes with a weak, 7 hertz electromagnetic field. 18 hours later, little pieces of DNA had grown in the original tube, which consisted of only pure sterilized water." (37)

The giant DNA molecule begins as a quantum wave

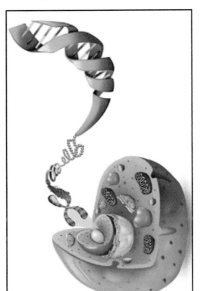

One strand of DNA from one single cell contains enough information to clone an entire organism. Obviously, understanding DNA allows us to understand much about life and the universe around us. A deeper understanding of the new science tells us that DNA begins not as a molecule, but as a wave form. "Even more interestingly, this wave form exists as a pattern within time and space and is coded throughout the entire universe." (37) As this wave turns into a particle it solidifies as molecule.

"We are surrounded by pulsating waves of invisible genetic information, whose waves create microscopic gravitational forces. They pull in atoms and molecules from their surrounding environment to construct the molecule DNA." (16)

Everywhere in the universe biological life is constantly in the process of creation, whenever and wherever it can. Micro gravitational waves will begin by gathering atoms and molecules to create DNA, and thus, creating life. (38)

Deep inside every cell of our body, protected by the nucleus, lays an organic macro-molecule, the DNA. It is the carrier of the genetic code. All genes responsible for the construction of our body and our whole life are generated in the DNA.

The molecule deoxyribonucleic acid (DNA) is one of nature's greatest masterpieces. It consists of two parallel strands of phosphate and sugar molecules, which are connected at regular intervals (of about three hundred millionths of an inch) by "ladder rungs," the so-called base pairs with each other. In general, a DNA molecule is like a giant zipper.

Crucial for the genetic information are the ladder rungs. They consist of only four nitrogen-containing chemicals called nucleotides or bases. These are adenine (A), thymine (T), cytosine (C) and guanine (G).

The Double Helix of the DNA

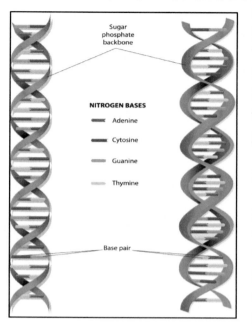

Only adenine and thymine or cytosine and guanine, form such a bridge together. There are only four possible combinations: A-T, T-A, C-G and G-C. The result is a very specific code, based on the arrangement and sequence of these base pairs along the DNA double strand. A unique signification can be derived out of these mere four letters A, T, C and G. Out of this code, all the genetic information of an organism is determined.

Stretched out, a DNA molecule would have a length of nearly two meters. "With our naked eyes we could still not see it, because it would be only about seven trillionth centimeters thick," says Grazyna Fosar, a pioneering scientist and journalist. To accommodate something so gigantic in the nucleus of every human cell, "the DNA simply rolls up into a ball. The double strand winds initially like a coil spring or double helix." This spins until it fits on a space of only about one billionth of a cubic centimeter. Genes are functional sections of DNA, each section serving a common purpose. Just imagine the human body contains 800 billion cells. This omnipotent DNA houses in virtually every cell. (39)

The Geno- and Phenotype

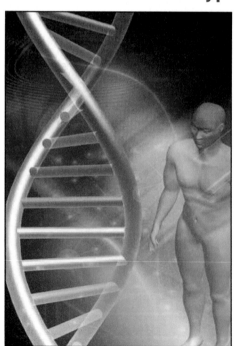

In this macromolecule, all information for development, function and individuality of any living being is encoded in an organized yet individual manner. Generally speaking the DNA is made up of two types, the geno- and the phenotype.

The genotype corresponds to the autonomous basic plan, which is the same for all living creatures of this type. This does not alter during the lifetime of an organism. For instance, it determines that this genome is specifically for the building blocks of a human being. All over this planet, a human being comes with one head, two arms, two legs, with certain organs and with certain functions. All this is coded information in the genotype part of DNA.

On the other hand, the phenotype expresses the interaction of the genotype with the environment, with social and socio-political influences, as well as personal sex, individual genetic affinities, attitudes, and thoughts. The phenotype is the sum of all the morphological, physiological, psychological and molecular characteristics of an individual. This includes individual experiences in wars, starvation, prosperity, beliefs or behavioral patterns.

This phenotype corresponds to the individual aspect of DNA. It is changeable. The Geno- and the Phenotype are inextricably combined.

The Human Genome

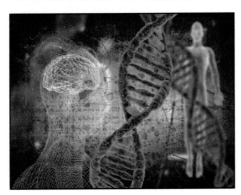

An organism's complete set of DNA is called its genome. Virtually every single cell in the body contains a complete copy of the approximately 3 billion DNA base pairs, or letters, that make up the human genome.

They reside in the 23 pairs of chromosomes within the nucleus of all our cells. Each chromosome contains hundreds to thousands of genes, which carry the instructions for making proteins. Each of the estimated 30,000 genes in the human genome makes an average of three proteins. (40)

The known genes account for only about 2 percent of the entire DNA molecule. The remaining 98 percent are for most modern geneticists, who consider only the biochemical side of the DNA, silent or even junk. A great percentage of our DNA molecule is not even involved in the actual heredity process.

Russian scientists pondered on this. Yes, they verified the fact, that roughly 90 percent of this DNA molecule is not responsible for protein synthesis. They discovered that an enormous part of the DNA molecule serves for communication and information purposes. Nothing in the human organism is useless or mute.

The DNA as rod and ring antenna
By the characteristic shape of the double helix, the DNA is an almost ideal electromagnetic antenna. "One part," says Grazyna Fosar "is elongated and thus a rod antenna which can receive very good electrical impulses. On the other hand, as seen from above, it looks like a ring. Therefore it is simultaneously a very good magnetic antenna." This enables the DNA to capture electromagnetic radiation. The energy is stored in the DNA by the molecule's own oscillation. (39) Prof. Dr. Popp confirmed their natural frequency lay at 150 megahertz. (41)

According to the research done by Pyotr Garjajev (42) and his team the "DNA is the transmitter and receiver of electromagnetic energy. It is also an interpreter of the information contained in the radiation." The two German physicists Grazyna Fosar and Franz Bludorf refer to the "DNA as a highly complex interactive biochip based on light with 4 gigabits of storage capability." Indeed, the DNA is even in a position to understand the human language. (39)

The DNA is mother of all languages
The Russian language researchers found that the genetic code follows the same rules as all our human languages. They compared the rules of syntax, the semantics, and the basic rules of grammar. Fosar und Bludorf translated scientific research papers from Russia and created in their

book *Networking Intelligence* a vivid picture, how DNA follows own regular grammar rules like in our language – and how it connects to our language. They indorse the scientific understanding "human languages did not appear by chance, but are a reflection of our innate DNA." The Russian biophysicist and molecular biologist Pyotr Garjajev and his colleagues also studied the vibrational behavior of DNA. In one experiment, they set the specific frequency patterns on a laser beam to influence the DNA frequency and thus the genetic information itself. Since the basic structure of the DNA alkaline pairs and the language are of the same structure, the decoding of the DNA was not required. (39)

Words and phrases of the human language can easily be used. Experiments have proven it frequently. "The code the DNA uses for communication can be described as the primal language of mankind and all beings in the universe", concludes Garjajev in his book.

Wormholes are communication channels

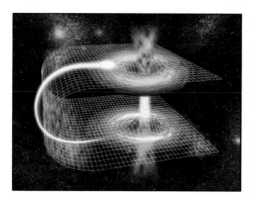

Modern biology, especially genetics, has long been involved with the study of the hereditary molecule, the DNA, the carrier of our genes. The Finnish scientist Matti Pitkänen (43) opens unimaginable possibilities with his brilliant theory. Communication takes place through magnetized wormholes. In 1957, the physicist John Wheeler described "wormholes as microscopic connecting channels through hyperspace caused by the quantum vacuum fluctuation". (44) According to Pitkänens theory, the magnetized wormholes accumulate at sequences of this huge DNA biomolecule and serve as communication channels.

A wormhole is a "tube made of space-time" that connects two different regions. If it's set up properly, you could enter one side of the tube and exit the other end somewhere else, or even at another time. Michio Kaku, in his book *A Scientific Odyssey through Parallel Universes, Time Warps, and the Tenth Dimension*, describes a wormhole tapering down a funnel to a 'throat,' which although thinner, never pinches off entirely. It connects to another funnel that opens up somewhere else. (45) Some people refer to them as shortcuts through the universe, while others claim they may be a means of traveling through time.

The DNA is used for communication

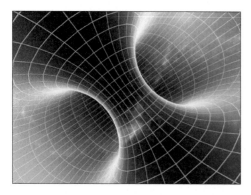

An interdisciplinary research group of the Russian Academy of Sciences in Moscow under the direction of the molecular biologist and biophysicist Dr. Pjotr P. Garjajev confirmed Pitkänens theory in research results. The communication in the DNA, the information storage and transmission takes place not in the classical way, but through magnetized wormholes. "This is space-time-free through the higher dimensions of hyper-space." John Staughton explains the wormholes in a more technical method by referring to them "as Einstein-Rosen bridges, as they were first proposed by Albert Einstein and Nathan Rosen in 1935. These bridges across space-time are believed to be possible due to the bending effect that all massive objects have on space-time." (46) The DNA attracts these bits of information and passes them on to our consciousness. (47)

Scientists discover photon tunneling in human brain

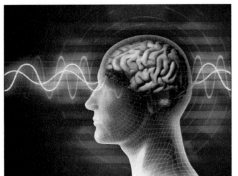

For Russian scientists wormholes are communication channels. More than 50 years later American scientists discovered similar channels and termed them "photon tunnels." In July 2016, a group of Canadian researchers from the University of Calgary and University of Alberta, discovered a fundamentally new type of communication between neurons in the brain. Neurons communicate via photon tunnels.

As experts explain, "the refractive index of myelin is higher than that of the intercellular environment, which theoretically allows it to pass through the photons. Thus, the myelin sheath and biophotons can form a quantum optical network in the brain."

"Biophotons, which are the result of oxidation reactions," according to the authors of this new study can be perfect information carriers, "since body temperature may influence the movement of electrical impulses, but not the propagation of light. Besides, the transmission of information via photons could be millions of times faster than what is believed today." (48)

Hypercommunication

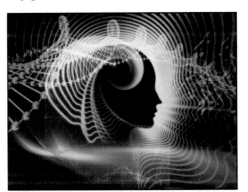

The two scientists, Fosar and Bludorf, compare the "DNA to sophisticated antennae, using the mysterious force of gravity as a bond to contain microscopic wormholes, which act like a fiber-optic network." Hyper-communication seems to be a perfect description of this process. "Incoming information and data is received by the DNA and then transmitted via the body's neural network to the brain. The brain, in turn, transforms it into very real human experiences, as they are often triggered during altered states of consciousness." (49) In expanding our awareness, we allow hypercommunication via quantum tunnels to be perceived. This "would be like unzipping and configuring a computer program, opened only when the correct mental stimulus is given."

This communication takes place outside of time and space on a higher dimensional hyperspace. (50) Hypercommunication describes situations when someone suddenly accesses information outside his or her personal knowledge base. Stress, anxiety, and a hyperactive brain cripple this ability. Fosar and Bludorf compare it with an intergalactic internet.

"Just like the Internet, the DNA
- feeds its own data in this network,
- retrieves data from the network and
- takes direct contact with other participants of the network."

In his book *Infinite Mindfield: A Quest to Find the Gateway to Higher Consciousness*, Anthony Peake explains the process used by DNA to stores information "by simply applying the principles of soliton waves." (51) In 1834, Scott Russel described the soliton phenomenon. A soliton is a single, well-defined wave that can travel great instances while maintaining its original shape. It acts as a carrier wave of the DNA. Hypercommunication is obviously neither subject to any restrictions nor even a certain specified purpose. It rather represents an interface to an open network - a consciousness or life network. (42)

"You can have your own 'homepage' so to speak, you can 'surf' the web and 'chat' with other participants," claims Grazyna Fosar. (39) The DNA is not, as one might perhaps believe, limited to their own species. Different creatures share the genetic information with each other in this way. The hypercommunication is therefore a first scientifically verifiable interface through which the different forms of intelligence of the universe are interconnected. (42) The skills of horse whisperers could also be explained with this theory.

Communication channels for a higher purpose

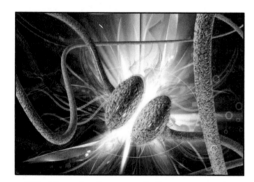

Who communicates and who has interest in human data? Is there anyone orchestrating this data? It gets exciting, especially since we know our DNA has the ability to communicate with data from other people, or more generally with other living beings. The DNA uses wormholes that dock right on the DNA molecule. (52) Could it be that these communication channels explicitly serve a higher essence that guides, organizes and gives life to this ball of light, the body? If we can imagine that, then it would take a higher form of existence to be involved with the design and the operation of this DNA.

The two physicists and mathematicians Grazyna Fosar and Franz Bludorf summarized breathtaking research results. They are convinced that "DNA is not only a biochemical factory. It has its own perceptual apparatus and can extend its probes far into any environment, beyond the limits of the body, even beyond space and time." (39)

Information from the future

Is it possible to communicate with far more advanced beings, higher life forms at another time, in another universe? Can we download schematics, musical creations, healing methods and simultaneously build a future to which we are then frequency-specific? Yes, science shows it.

In 1965 Paul McCartney was staying at his parent's house. "I woke up with a lovely tune in my head. I thought, 'That's great, I wonder what that is?' There was a piano next to me, to the right of the bed by the window. I got out of bed, sat at the piano, found G, found F sharp minor 7th -- and that lead me through then to B to E minor, and finally back to E. It all lead forward logically. I liked the melody a lot, but because I'd dreamed it, I couldn't believe I'd written it. I thought, 'No, I've never written anything like this before.' But I had the tune, which was the most magic thing!" The tune McCartney was speaking about turned out to be the gigantic hit *Yesterday*.

In 1997, the song was inducted into the Grammy Hall of Fame. The *Guinness Book of Records* holds that *Yesterday* is the most covered song ever with over 3000 versions recorded, and Broadcast Music Incorporated asserts the song was performed over seven million times in the 20th century alone... all from a dream. (53)

The great philosopher and mathematician Bertrand Russel frankly admits that he could solve many of his difficult problems with the help of his dreams. More examples of dream solutions are the structure of the periodic system from Dimitri Mendeleyev, the structure of the atom from physicist Niels Bohr and the mass production of insulin by Sir Frederick Banting.

Johannes Brahms wrote, "I see not only certain themes before my mind's eye, but also the right form in which they are dressed, the harmony and the orchestration. The finished work is revealed to me by measure." August Kekulé found the structure formula of benzene during a nightmare and Nikola Tesla had his inspiration during the walk on how to build an alternating current generator. (53)

In humans, hyper-communication can mostly be seen as:
- Clairvoyance
- Intuition, inspiration
- Spontaneous and remote acts of healing
- Self-healing

In nature hyper-communication is an applied and proven concept for millions of years. It ensures an orderly flow of life as demonstrated in insect societies.

Hypercommunication in an ant-colony

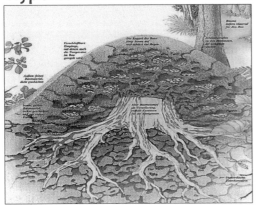

For some creatures, like ants, hypercommunication is a natural part of daily business. When a queen ant is spatially separated from her colony her subjects continue to work and build fervently and according to plan. If she's killed, however, the ants become aimless and all work instantly halts. Apparently, as long as the queen ant is alive, she can communicate with the group consciousness of her colony through means of hypercommunication. She can be as far away as she wants, as long as she is alive. (54)

The biologist Rupert Sheldrake speaks about morphic fields. Morphic fields of social groups connect members of the group even when they are many miles apart, and provide clear channels of communication, even at enormous distances. Science knows of telepathic abilities of many species. Telepathy seems to be normal means of animal communication.

In his book *Dogs That Know When Their Owners Are Coming Home* Sheldrake gives some examples: How does a dog know when its owner is returning home at an unexpected time? How do cats know when it is time to go to the vet, even before the cat carrier comes out? How do horses find their way back to the stable over completely unfamiliar terrain? And how can some pets predict that their owners are about to have an epileptic fit? (55)

The DNA and Wave Genetics

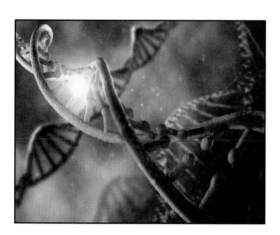

Genes in the DNA are influenced by certain resonant electro-magnetic waves. This process is called wave genetics.

In applying wave genetics Russian scientists performed genetic alterations without the known dangers of conventional genetics. Fosar and Bludorf document some of their successful experiments "to repair genes by stimulating cancer cells for self-healing. The 'remedies' in this case were not medicines, but information. To feed this medicinal information into the DNA, the DNA code does not have to be deciphered. The DNA responds to our own words of our daily language." (39) Peter Garjajev, Director of Wave Genetics Institute in Moscow is convinced that the immense power of wave genetics is unfolding "with greater influence on the formation of organisms than the biochemical processes of alkaline information or intent. This wave energy will create reality." (56)

The DNA as a Fractal

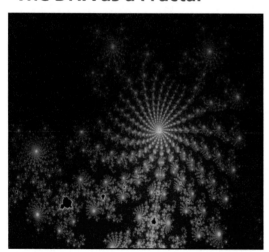

Fractals are one of the most fundamental concepts in nature. Their Role was discovered by Benoit Mandelbrot in 1975. Fractals are neither lines nor surfaces, but infinitely complex, self-similar structures, which are repeated both in large as in small.

"In the genetic DNA code, the structure of the enveloping soliton wave occurs in numerous repetitions and self-similarities," as Pyotr Garjajev emphasized. This means that the information in the DNA is not read in linear sequences, like you read a book. "Instead, the reading operation is carried out forward and backward, upward and downward, it sometimes also returns to the starting point." (57)

Scientist at Princeton University discovered that "nonlinear systems supporting solitons can often, (under proper conditions,) give rise to self-similarity and fractals on successively smaller scales. Such fractals can be observed in most soliton-supporting systems in nature." (58) The information pattern the DNA receives is stored in a soliton wave. The DNA communication follows fractal laws. It takes place non-locally. Garjajev is convinced that, "the DNA may also communicate with remote information carriers without being bound by time and space. This communication travels by the speed of light. This effect goes back to a famous paradox of science, the so-called Einstein-Podolsky-Rosen paradox." This states that two particles of matter, which were joined and were then separated, remain connected to each other forever. If one of these two particles changes, the other responds instantly, even if the two particles are light years away from each other. (59)

A study published in 2011 comes to the conclusion: "The wide frequency range of interaction with EMF (electromagnetic field) is the functional characteristic of a fractal antenna, and DNA appears to possess the two structural characteristics of fractal antennas, electronic conduction and symmetry. These properties contribute to greater reactivity of DNA with EMF in the environment, and the DNA damage could account for increases in cancer epidemiology." (60)

With this new understanding of non-locality communication the law of cause and effect was broken. Garjajev writes, "Cause and effect are not separated by time. Time can be understood as a way of organizing a chain event. This requires a complicated fractal structure of time, which is the reason why it was unrecognized by Einstein." (61)

According to Garjajev, this quantum non-locality plays a key function in the self-organization of living matter. There are also non-physical forms of communication, e.g. telepathy. (62)

The phantom DNA Effect

The most incredible part of Dr. Garjajev's experiment came when he thought the experiment was over. Edward Morgan talks about a very extraordinary experiment when Garjajev "pulled a DNA strand from the quartz container and looked back into the container only to find that photons were still spiraling in the exact same place where the DNA had been. Apparently, some sort of gravitational influence was holding photons right where the DNA had been." Scientists term this phenomenon the "DNA phantom effect." It seems that an energetic force being created by the DNA absorbs photons and pulls them right into the DNA molecule. The DNA as matter is not needed anymore. "The invisible force field attracts and holds the light (photons) there all by itself." (16)

Dr. Garjajev found that "he could blast the phantom with super cold liquid nitrogen gas and the photons would escape from the force field. After 5 to 8 minutes though, new photons would resurface and the entire phantom would reappear. He could keep doing this as much as he wanted, but new photons would keep appearing. In fact, it was only after doing this for 30 days straight that the photons finally did not reappear." (16)

The effect can be repeated at any given time. The scientific explanation explains that apparently the DNA itself generates a noise pattern in a vacuum. These patterns in the vacuum, caused by the presence of living matter, can continue for several months in extreme cases.

The Russian research group under Pyotr Garjajev proved that chromosomes, which were damaged for example by X-rays, were repaired. In another experiment, the researchers used informational patterns of a particular DNA and inserted them into another DNA. Thus, they reprogrammed cells to another genome. (63)

Man is the creator of his own reality

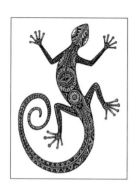

Russian scientist Dr. Peter Garjajev discovered that DNA absorbs light photons in its surrounding area. Knowing that this spiraling communication effect continues for up to 30 days, he started a new experiment. "Garjajev directed a gentle laser beam through a developing salamander embryo and redirected it into a developing frog embryo. This caused the frog embryo's DNA to completely re-code itself with the instructions to build a healthy adult salamander, even though the two embryos were in hermetically sealed containers and only light was allowed to pass through." (64) Fosar and Bludorf use the outcome to demonstrate the implications for many fields of medicine and genetics.

Multiple strand DNA

The human race as of today knows very little about itself, almost like a race in amnesia. As we continue to move forward through time, new discoveries are made that make old theories obsolete and false.

In 2012, about sixty years after the discovery of the double helix, scientists identified quadruplex DNA strands in human cancer cells. Quadruple helices intertwine four, rather than two strands of DNA. The four-stranded packages of DNA, called G-quadruplexes, are formed by the interaction of four guanine bases that together make a square. "They appear to be transitory structures, and are most abundant when the cells are poised to divide. They originate in chromosomes and in telomeres. Telomeres are the caps on the tips of chromosomes that protect them from damage." (65) The discovery was published online in *Nature Chemistry*, Jan 2012. The study was led by Shankar Balasubramanian at the University of Cambridge, UK. (66)

April 2011, the first child with 3-strand DNA is born

A two-year-old boy was the first recorded person in the world to be diagnosed with an extra strand in his DNA. Such children are clairvoyant and can converse telepathically.

Doctors revealed "his seventh chromosome had an extra strand of material which had never been documented anywhere in the world before." (67)

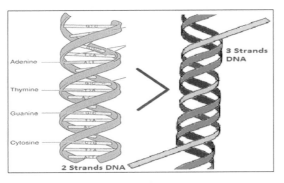

Source: www.humansarefree.com

The question is how many DNA strands can human beings possess? Some geneticists are claiming humans will have 13 strands one day.

The Pulse of the DNA

The DNA pulsates, it vibrates. In rhythmic cycles it contracts and expands again. During this process, the DNA stores and emits light. The same pulsation takes place in all natural large and small systems, organisms or their components, actually in the entire seen and unseen world. The prevailing principle of contraction and expansion, of exhaling and inhaling, attraction and repulsion, involution and evolution is omnipresent in nature. (59)

Pierre Franckh, in his book *The DNA Field and the Law of Resonance* describes that "cells are in a constant interaction with sunlight and accumulate coherence through this process. The resulting field can store more and longer wave frequencies by enclosing them in its structure. Thus, the cell becomes an increasingly better resonator. It expands its communications base, its possibilities to exchange information, but also the opportunity to build a complex organism with other cells." (68)

The authors Grazyna Fosar and Franz Bludorf explain these actions explicitly in their book *Vernetzte Intelligenz (Networking Intelligence)*. (39)

The DNA masterplan
The DNA contains the masterplan for the creation of proteins and other molecules and systems of the cell. It contains all of the instructions a cell needs to sustain itself. These instructions are found within genes, which are sections of DNA made up of specific sequences of nucleotides. In order to be implemented, the instructions contained within genes must be expressed, or copied into a form that can be used by cells to produce the proteins needed to support life.

RNA, the copying agents
The instructions stored in the DNA are read and processed by a cell in two steps: transcription and translation. Each step is a separate biochemical process involving multiple molecules. "During transcription, a portion of the cell's DNA serves as a template for the creation of an RNA molecule. In some cases, the newly created RNA molecule is the finished product, and it serves an important function within the cell. In other cases, the RNA molecule carries messages from the DNA to other parts of the cell for processing." Predominantly, this information is used to manufacture

proteins. The specific type of RNA that carries the information stored in DNA to other areas of the cell is called messenger RNA, or mRNA. (69)

Transcription begins when an enzyme called RNA polymerase attaches to the DNA template strand and begins assembling a new chain of nucleotides to produce a complementary RNA strand. There are multiple types of types of RNA.

Transcription factors support as well the selection which DNA sequences should be transcribed as the precise order in which this transcription process should take place. The most prevalent protein in this process is the large enzyme Polymerase. (69)

It is obvious, that errors in DNA replication can cause serious consequences. If the DNA is not correctly replicated, the cell will not perform its intended function. (70)

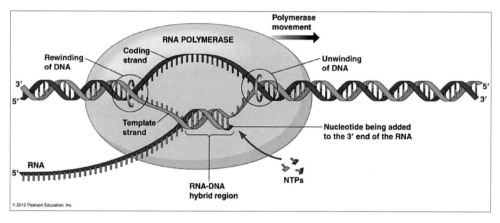

Source: 2012 Pearson Education Inc.

What or who is the mastermind behind this masterplan? And where is the energy source for these extreme exact functioning processes coming from?

Light is the organizing principle of matter

With its structure and its dimensions, the DNA is the ideal antenna, the ideal resonator for visible sunlight. Thus, the distance of its base pairs corresponds exactly to the ability of sunlight to release its power in the cell.

The Sun and Vitamin D

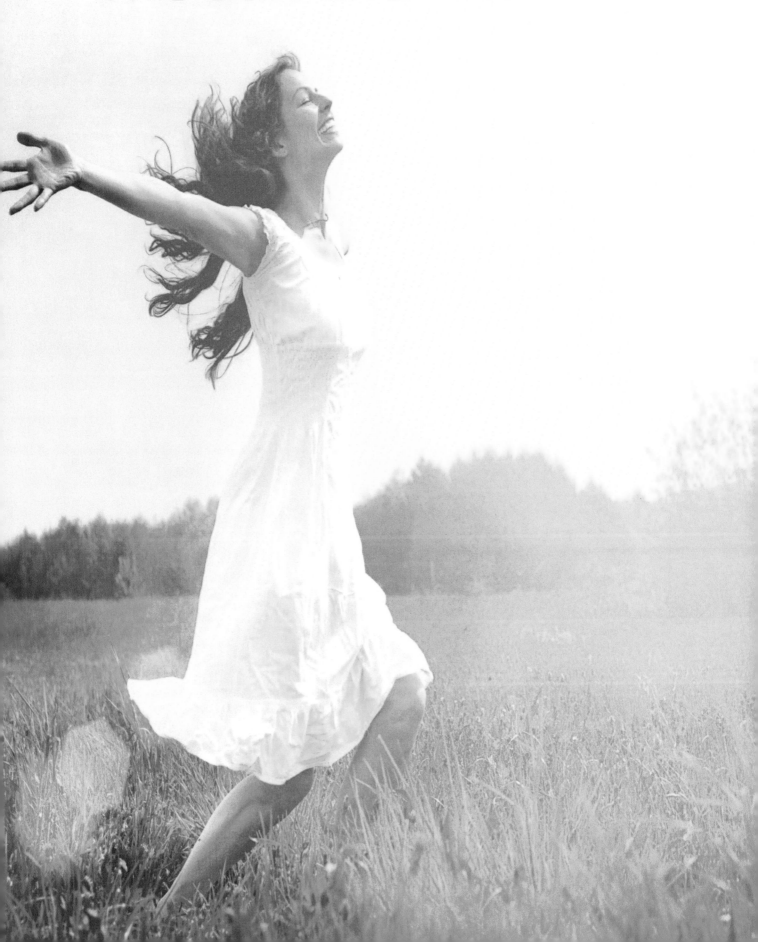

Chapter Three

Sun's Healing Power and Vitamin D

"Beautifully you appear in the horizon of heaven, living sun that determines life! You have risen in the eastern horizon and have filled every country with your beauty. You are beautiful, great and bright, high above all the land." (Canticle to the sun of Pharaoh Akhenaton)

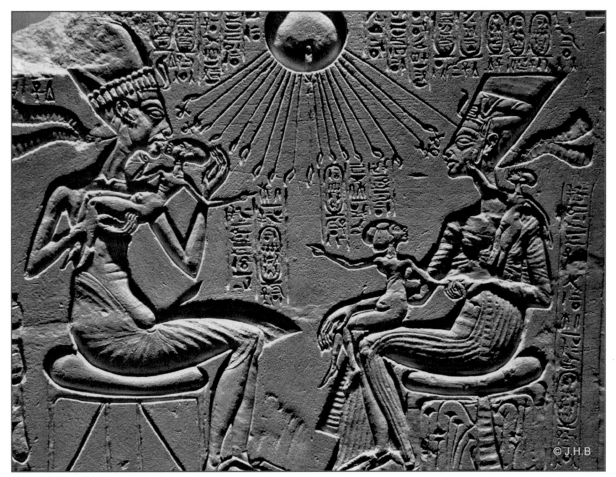

Source: https://commons.wikimedia.org

Pharaoh Akhenaton described a cornerstone of his belief of light, the sun, "The path of the sun guarantees the continuity of the world and the cosmos. Every day the sun god renews his creation. Moreover, as he descends each night into the underworld, he brings the dead back to life. There, in the underworld, he regenerates and overcomes the dangers of darkness and chaos."

The sun is the greatest energy generator and energy source. Vitamin D is recognized as the sunshine vitamin. It has been produced on this earth through sunlight for more than 500 million years. From an evolutionary perspective, phytoplankton and zooplankton existed in our oceans for over 500 million years producing vitamin D when exposed to sunlight.

Vitamin D – a powerful molecule

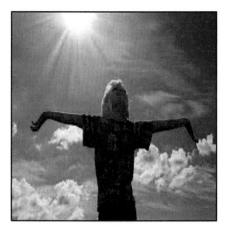

The skin is one of the largest human organs. With an area of one and a half to two square meters and with 15 percent of the body weight it is the largest sensory organ of the human body. It produces vitamin D through sun exposure. It is the cell membrane that stimulates the biophoton activity through certain aspects of sunlight.

World renowned cell biologist Bruce Lipton (71) confirms, "The true secret of life lies exactly at the interface between the inside and the outside of a cell, and this cell membrane is just a tiny little seven millionths of a millimeter thick. This cellular membrane skin is used by our body to convert environmental signals of behavior. In the same way as our nervous system functions the membrane proteins control and govern all life processes of the cell." Here in the membranogenic lipids, the fatty acids of the membrane are the starting point of the vitamin D synthesis. (72)

Vitamin D3 is the only vitamin our body builds by itself - all that is needed is direct sunlight and the skin.

The Sun - DNA - and vitamin D

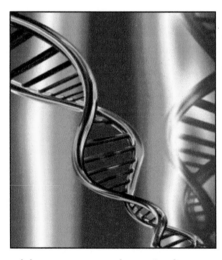

Sunlight supports life on this planet. All planetary life vibrates with a DNA frequency specific to the sun. Sunlight pulsates; it contracts in a rhythmic undulation and expands like the DNA. Through this pulsating process vitamin D can be produced in almost every cell. This creates an ongoing strong atmospheric field. The cell is pulsating while the DNA absorbs the light particles. A biophotonic absorption, processing, exchange, storing and transmitting is taking place.

Vitamin D is the carrier of information. Vitamin D is regarded as a kind of "super hormone." In fact, it is formed from cholesterol like the steroid hormones, estrogen, testosterone, progesterone, aldosterone and cortisol.

JZ Knight, the inventor of the Blu Room, and Dr. Matthew Martinez, her co-developer, lovingly call Vitamin D the "God-hormone."

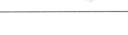

History of vitamin D and light therapy

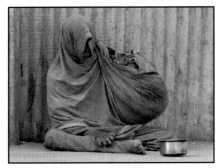

In the Middle Ages

Leprosy is an infectious bacterial disease, which affects the skin, mucous membranes and nerve cells. The causative agent of leprosy disease is mycobacterium leprae. In the Middle Ages the diagnosis leprosy was equal to a death sentence for a person. He was then thrown out of human society as a leper. Covered with a white sheet from head to toe the person was carried to church on a stretcher. A Requiem was read in the presence of the community. Then he was wrapped in thicker garments including a hood and was sent as a leper to permanent settlement far outside the village. This meant a miserable and painfully short life. Whoever rejected this procedure was sent out stark naked into the uncivilized desert or the forest. He lived in the fields, exposed to the sun and the wind and often came back after months in a healthy condition.

The industrial revolution

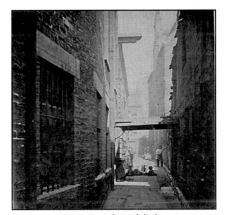

Source: Open Book Publishers

The first evidence of the importance of sunlight for human health began with the industrial revolution in northern Europe in the 1600s. People were living in huge blocks built in close vicinity to each other. The burning of coal and wood polluted the atmosphere. Yet it was this industry which gave many people hope and livelihood. Many of the people moved from rural villages into newly built apartment blocks. The children had very little exposure to sunlight. Soon physicians observed that these children had growth retardation and skeletal deformities, including bony projections along the rib cage and either bowed legs or knocked knees. They called this disease rickets. (73)

Children in the United States, i.e. New York City and Boston were raised in a similar polluted sunless environment. They too developed rickets.

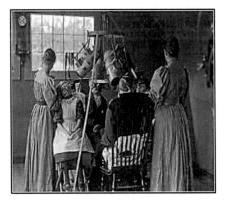

Source: Finsen Institute Copenhagen

The first phototherapy

In 1877 Downes and Blunt proved that sunlight exerts a bactericidal action and could kill anthrax bacilli. In 1890 Palm from Edinburgh suggested that the sun could play a therapeutic role in rickets. (74)

In 1896 Niels Ryberg Finsen, the father of ultraviolet therapy, developed a bacteria-destroying lamp. With this "Finsen Lamp" he treated over 800 patients with lupus vulgaris in his Phototherapy

Institute in Copenhagen. Documents report a cure of 80 percent. (75)

In 1903, Finsen was awarded the Nobel Prize in medicine "in recognition for the treatment of lupus vulgaris, with concentrated light rays". (75)

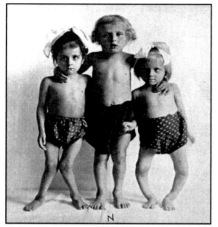

Source: commons.wikimedia.org/wiki

Sun exposure as therapy

In the 19th century, sunlight became progressively more significant for medical purposes. In 1822, Śniadecki a Polish physician, chemist and biologist was the first to document the possible relationship between the industrialization of Northern Europe and rickets. He reported of children living in the inner city of Warsaw having a high incidence of rickets due to their lack of sun exposure. Contrarily, he observed that children living in rural areas outside of Warsaw did not suffer from rickets.

Śniadecki wrote "the sun must be regarded as the most efficient method for the prevention and cure of this disease". (73) The Royal Infirmary in Manchester used cod liver oil to heal rickets.

Soon ultraviolet lamps were available. In the winter of 1918/1919 Huldschinsky, a German pediatrician, successfully demonstrated how rickets could be treated with ultra-violet lamps. At that time perhaps half of all German children suffered from rickets. It was already recognized that this disease was caused by calcium deficiency due to lack of sunlight. Thereafter heliotherapy was a common practice for many illnesses.

The *Bonekey Report* published in 2014 presents detailed information of the history of rickets before discovery of vitamin D. "Progress in studies of the causes and treatment of rickets suddenly moved much faster, in the period 1917–1922. At the beginning of that time, Huldschinsky recommended ultraviolet light treatment for rickets. At the same time, Hess showed that cod liver oil could prevent and cure rickets in Afro-American children in New York." In 1921 Hess and Unger (76) exposed rachitic children to sunlight on the roof of their hospital in New York City and demonstrated significant improvements in the children's health. These physicians also realized that children of darker pigmented skin were at much higher risk for rickets. They concluded that dark skinned children needed longer exposure to sunlight to both treat and prevent rickets. (77)

In 1920s Walter H. Ude MD of Minneapolis General Hospital reported a "series of 100 cases in which he claimed an almost 100 percent cure rate with ultraviolet skin irradiation." (78)

This method was abandoned with the advent of the antibiotic revolution.

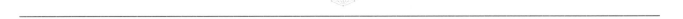

The discovery of vitamin D

Vitamin D was first isolated from tuna fish oil in 1936, and consequently synthesized in 1952. Vitamin D3 (Cholecalciferol) is the form humans and other animals produce. It is also found in fish liver oil. Fish get their vitamin D initially in the food chain from planktonic algae. Big fish eat little fish, and we eat them.

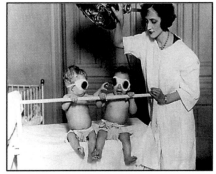

The research group around McCollum (79) concluded that the substance curing rickets is a new vitamin. They called it vitamin D (alphabetically named 'D' as the fourth known vitamin). In additional papers published in 1924 Hess and other researchers described (80) the effects of the ultraviolet irradiation of food. Thus the scene was set for the remarkable progress that followed the discovery of vitamin D.

Source: www.worthytoshare.com

The United States government also established an agency in 1931 whose goal was to promote sensible sun exposure of young children to prevent rickets and improve their bone health.

Vitamin D became so popular that in the 1930s and 1940s a wide variety of foods and beverages as well as personal care products were fortified with vitamin D. (81) They included not only milk and other dairy products but also soda pop, beer, hot dogs, custard and even soap and shaving cream.

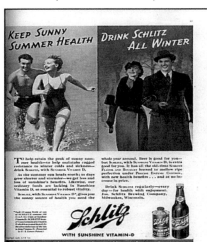

In 1936, Schlitz even promoted their vitamin D fortified beer in wintertime with the slogan "Keep sunny summer health all winter long - drink vitamin D fortified Schlitz beer." (82)

Carnation Milk also gained popularity through its innovation of irradiated evaporated milk. Irradiation involved exposing milk to ultraviolet rays produced by a quartz mercury lamp, and resulted in milk fortified with vitamin D. This milk fortified with vitamin D was the perfect solution for mothers reluctant to give their children daily doses of smelly, poor-tasting cod-liver oil. (83)

Source: American Magazine 1936

Since 1965 the importance of sun exposure and vitamin D in preventing and healing genetic, physical and mental disorders is widely documented. About 183 different diseases are related to the lack of sun exposure, ranging from diabetes type 1, hypertension, breast cancer, gingivitis, influenza, rickets, pregnancy risks, sickle cells, gestational diabetes, multiple sclerosis, depression, asthma, fibromyalgia, weight loss, congestive heart failure, Parkinson's disease, dementia, cystic fibrosis, Raynaud's syndrome, hip fractures, aging, prostate cancer, Crohn's disease, allergies, obesity and more. (84)

The lifesaving role of natural vitamin D and sunlight therapy lost attraction due to the appearance of antibiotics.

The Antibiotics Revolution
The era of antibacterial treatment began with the discoveries of arsenic-derived synthetic antibiotics by Alfred Bertheim and Paul Ehrlich in 1907. While their early compounds were too toxic, Ehrlich and Sahachiro Hata, a Japanese bacteriologist coworker succeeded with a new formed less toxic substance. The Hoechst Company began to market this compound toward the end of 1910 under the name Salvarsan.

In 1928 Sir Alexander Fleming discovered enzyme lysozyme and the antibiotic substance penicillin from the fungus Penicillium notatum. (85)

During the 1940's and 50's streptomycin, chloramphenicol, and tetracycline were discovered. In 1942 Selman Waksman used the term "antibiotics" to describe these compounds. The word antibiotic is derived from the Greek word "anti" which means "against," and "bios" meaning "life." Antibiotics transformed modern medicine.

Sunlight and its frequencies

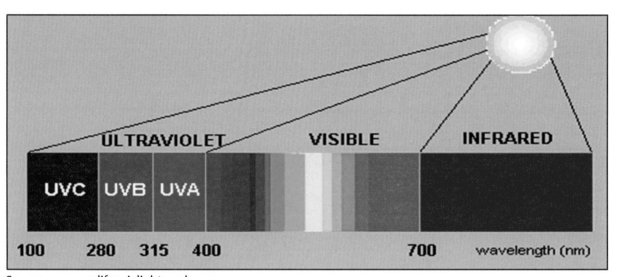

Source: www.californialightworks.com

Sunlight is a portion of the electromagnetic radiation given off by the sun, in particular infrared, visible, and ultraviolet light. On Earth, sunlight is filtered through the Earth's atmosphere, and is obviously perceived as daylight when the sun is above the horizon. UV radiation from the sun has always played important roles in our environment, and affects all living organisms. UV radiation at different wavelengths differs in its effects.

There are three forms of UV radiation that reach the Earth's surface, UVA, UVB and UVC. UVB has lower wavelength than UVA but higher energy.

Ultraviolet B or (UVB) range spans 280 to 315 nm. It is a medium wave radiation. It is also greatly absorbed by the Earth's atmosphere, and along with UVC causes the photochemical reaction leading to the production of the ozone layer. It is essential for vitamin D synthesis in the skin and fur of mammals. Every single molecule in human body, especially the DNA absorbs UVB radiation very efficiently.

Ultraviolet A or (UVA) spans 315 to 400 nm. It is a long wave radiation. UVA radiation is not absorbed as efficiently, so it penetrates deep into the dermis and can cause skin damage, including cross-linking of the collagen matrix. A great deal of immunosuppression occurs in the UVA range, for example the formation of free radicals and reactive oxygen species.

The spectrum of the sunlight UVA, UVB and UVC (short wave) radiation occurs naturally as a component of sunlight, and is referred to as ultraviolet light.

UVA Radiation	UVB Radiation
Direct tanning lasts only hours	Delayed, long lasting tan
No skin protection by pigmentation	Excellent vitamin D production
Causes skin aging	No skin aging
Produces large quantities of free radicals	Virtually no production of free radicals

Only the UVB radiation from the sun is responsible for the production of vitamin D. Both wavelengths differ in their effect.

Excessive exposure to UVA radiation produces large amounts of free radicals and causes genetic disorders of irradiated skin cells. Usually this genetic damage can be easily corrected by the endogenous repair systems – yet if the radiation is in excess, a risk of skin cancer may ensue.

Ultraviolet light has shorter wave lengths than visible light. Though these waves are invisible to human eye, some insects like the bumble bees can see them.

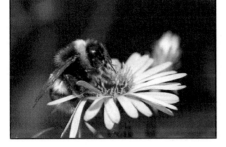

Bees have remarkable eyesight. Nobel Prize-winning scientist Karl von Frisch discovered honey bees' secret language. Frisch proved that bees have the ability to see color based on their perception of UV light. Humans may see more colors, yet bees have a much broader range of color vision. Their ability to see ultraviolet light gives them an advantage when seeking nectar. (86)

Other scientists also assume that ultraviolet vision in bees might the source of their social interactions or communication.

Factors influence the ability to produce vitamin D

Sun induced vitamin D synthesis is greatly influenced by season, time of day, latitude, altitude, air pollution, skin pigmentation, sunscreen use, passing through glass and plastic, clothes and individual situations.

Seasons of the year and latitude

Only about one percent of solar UVB radiation reaches the Earth's surface even during summer at noon time. The reason is that all of the UVC (200–280 nm) and all of the UVB radiation up to approximately 290nm are efficiently absorbed by the stratospheric ozone layer. The ozone layer also absorbs approximately 99% of the UVB radiation with wavelengths 291–315 nm. The path of solar UVB is lengthened through the ozone layer. Naturally the number of UVB photons that reach the Earth's surface is reduced. (87)

It is a well-known fact that in winter very little if any vitamin D3 can be produced in the skin from sun exposure for people living above and below approximately 33° latitude. People who live farther North and South often cannot make any vitamin D3 in their skin for up to 6 month of the year. For example, in Boston at 42° North essentially no vitamin D3 can be produced in the skin from November through February. People living in Edmonton Canada at 52° North or Ushuaia Argentina at 55° South are unable to produce any significant vitamin D3 for about 6 month of the year. (88)

Generally, Vitamin D is produced in the skin exclusively between 10am and 3pm in the months of May until early September. In the early morning and late afternoon, the sun's rays are more oblique and get absorbed by the ozone layer. As a result, vitamin D is not produced in the skin.

Given the variations in latitude in the United States that may contribute to differences in sun exposure, studies reveal a link between allergic diseases and the various geographic environments. (89)

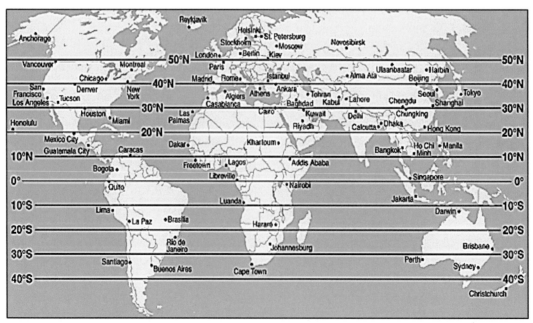

Altitude matters

Altitude can also have a dramatic influence on the amount of solar UVB that reaches the Earth's surface. The higher the altitude the shorter the path that UVB has to travel and thus the skin can produce more vitamin D3.

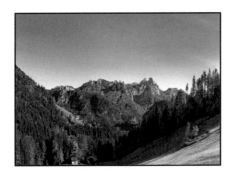

Since the beginning of the 20th century preferred areas for heliotherapy were established in the high mountains of Switzerland. People living below 1.600 meters altitude had a higher risk for tuberculosis, than people living in higher regions.

As early as 1842, the English physician Dr. John Davy had suggested that a mountain climate was likely to offer the best chances against tuberculosis, as "alpine people rarely had tubercles because of the greater respiratory activity occasioned by a rarified atmosphere." (90)

Reflectivity of the Earth's Surface

As a highly reflective substance, snow dramatically increases UVB exposure near the Earth's surface. Fresh snow can reflect much as 94 percent of the incoming UV radiation. In contrast, snow-free lands typically reflect only 2-4 percent of UV and ocean surfaces reflect about 5-8 percent. (91)

Aerosols and air pollution

Unlike clouds, aerosols in the troposphere, such as dust and smoke, not only scatter but also absorb UVB radiation. Usually the UV reduction by aerosols is only a few percent, but in regions of heavy smoke or dust, aerosol particles can absorb more than 50 percent of the radiation.

Dr. Michael Holick, the leading authority on vitamin D reports of the interference of air pollution and aerosols with the vitamin synthesis. "Additionally, widespread air pollution interferes with the vitamin D synthesis in two almost paradoxical ways. Particulate pollution reduces the amount of sunlight people receive, and ozone depletion causes people to minimize exposure to what sunlight there is. As people cover their skin to avoid skin cancer, they reduce their beneficial vitamin D production." (92)

Skin Pigmentation

Skin pigmentation was important in the evolution of humans as they migrated North and South of the equator. It is logical that heavily pigmented skin blocks up to 95% of UV radiation to the deepest skin layers. A decrease in the amount of skin pigment results in a decrease in the sun screening protection. More of the UVB radiation reaches the epidermal cells. Generally this applies to people with Caucasian origin.

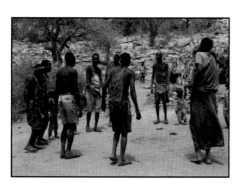

Africans such as the Maasai are exposed to sunlight throughout the year. The Maasai are no longer hunter-gatherers but live, along with their cattle, either a settled or a semi-nomadic lifestyle. They wear sparse clothes, which mainly cover their upper legs and upper body, and attempt to avoid the sun during the hottest part of the day. They eat mainly milk and meat from their cattle, although recently they began to add corn to their diet. Studies showed their major circulating form of vitamin D, 25(OH)D in the range of 46 ng/ml. (93)

Sunscreen and its effect

Natural sunscreen melanin

The skin has its own protection against radiation through sunlight. Keratinocytes are the most important of the epidermal cells. They produce a fibrous protein that gives the skin its protective properties. Melanocytes and keratinocytes work together in protecting the skin from UV damage. The role of the keratinocytes is to accumulate the melanin granules. The resulting pigment protects the DNA from UV radiation. Packets of body-generated sunscreen called melanin rise up into the epidermis and begin to coat all of the very important, sensitive components of the cell. (94) By doing so the beautiful tan works as a very effective sunscreen.

Melanin determines skin and hair color. Melanin is present in the skin to varying degrees depending on how much a population has been exposed to the sun historically.

Man-made synthetic sunscreens

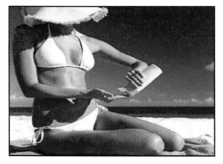

In the 1970s sunscreens flushed the market. Prevention of sunburn or even skin cancer was the first argument. The sunscreens contained UVB absorbing chemicals such as para-aminobenzoic acid. Researchers believed that only UVB radiation damages the skin and causes skin cancer. In-depth studies demonstrate that, "UVA radiation not only alters the immune system making it more immunotolerant but also increases the risk for non-melanoma and melanoma skin cancers." (89)

Sunscreen factors

Sunscreens were designed to absorb solar UVB radiation. A sunscreen with a sun protection factor (SPF) of 30 absorbs approximately 95–98 percent of solar UVB radiation. Hence a sunscreen with a protection factor of 30 reduces the capacity of the skin to produce vitamin D3 by the same amount. (95) A report confirmed "that the application of sunscreen with a SPF of only 8 dramatically reduced the blood level of vitamin D3 after exposure to sunlight." (96)

Mankind survived thousands of years without sunscreen. Our grandparents and great grandparents were mostly working outdoors. Sunscreen at that time was only for the high society. Our ancestors

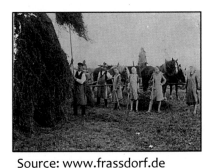

Source: www.frassdorf.de

lived and ate healthily. Skin cancer was hardly known. How would humans have made it this far without sunscreen for all those centuries if the sun was so dangerous?

Overexposure of sunlight

Overexposure to UV radiation in the whole spectrum of sunlight may cause harmful effects on the skin. Yet, no matter how much sun exposure a person has, it will never cause vitamin D intoxication because sunlight also destroys any excess vitamin D and previtamin D. (97) In addition, the body's own vitamin D is DNA frequency specific to this individual. Even when ingesting up to 1 million IUs of vitamin D3 daily for several months there was not one report of vitamin D intoxication. Vitamin D levels of 25(OH)D in blood serum showed > 500 ng/ml. This of course is not recommended and is associated with disorder of the calcium metabolism.

Under optimal conditions, fifteen minutes of sun exposure on face, hands and arms is sufficient for most people for a vitamin D production of about 10,000 IU. People with dark skin, obesity, tight clothing, and of certain age require different exposure times.

Studies have shown that the body of an adult with 70 kg body weight generates between 10,000 and 20,000 IU during a 20 minute sun tanning session. In the Blu Room, it takes only three minutes to generate this amount.

The metabolism of vitamin D

Until a few years ago it was believed, the active form of vitamin D is exclusively generated by the skin, liver and kidneys from sunlight.

The American researcher Prof. Michael F. Holick, professor of medicine, dermatology, physiology and biophysics discovered that every single cell in the body has the ability to form active vitamin D. Even in sunless times the body's DNA can generate its own vitamin D. "The healthier the cell is the more active the vitamin D generation is." (98)

The term vitamin D refers to two very similar molecules:
- Calciferol (D3), this is generated by ultraviolet radiation in human skin.
- Ergocalciferol (D2), this is found in certain foods.

Both pass through a multistage enzymatic conversion process to the biologically active form of 1,25-dihydroxycholecalciferol vitamin-D (Calcitriol).

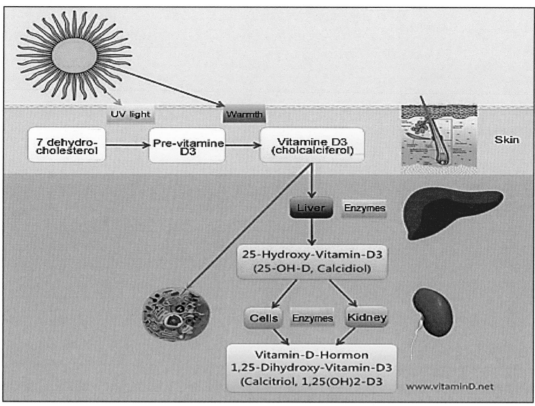

Source: www.vitaminD.net

The skin is able to manufacture not only vitamin D, but also has the enzymes to convert it into 25-Hydroxy vitamin D3 (25-OH-D or calcidiol) and finally to 1,25-dihydroxycholecalciferol vitamin D (Calcitriol). Several other types of tissue and immune cells can synthesize the enzyme that hydroxylates calcidiol to the active calcitriol.

- Vitamin D3 is constructed by certain skin cells keratinocytes, when the UVB radiation is applied to a degradation product of cholesterol, 7-dehydrocholesterol. These molecules move into the bloodstream.
- While circulating in the blood D3 passes through the liver, where enzymes convert it in 25-OH-Vitamin D3 (calcidiol).
- The kidneys proceed and convert 25-OH-Vitamin D3 through enzymatic reaction to finally result in the biologically active form 1,25-dihydroxycholecalciferol vitamin D (calcitriol).
- This complete process is governed by the body's own DNA. The produced vitamin D is fully accepted and put to use by the body.

This perfect molecule passes through the bloodstream to various organs, cell types and the DNA. 1,25-dihydroxycholecalciferol vitamin D plays an important role in regulating calcium and phosphate metabolism and controlling cell metabolism and genetic operations. Most cells and organs in the body have a vitamin D receptor and many cells and organs are able to produce 1,25-dihydroxycholecalciferol vitamin D. 25-OH vitamin D3 is the form that is circulating in the blood and also the value measured in blood tests. Vitamin D shows the best efficiency in blood levels between 30 and 80 ng /ml.

Vitamin D and its effects in the human body

Vitamin D controls more than 2,000 genes and thus has profound influence on the function of cells, organs and whole systems. (99) The effects of vitamin D are evident throughout the whole body and its design.

- Effects on the DNA
- Effects on the mineral balance
- Effects on the immune system
- Effects on the heart and circulation
- Effects on nerves and brain
- Effects on metabolism
- "Apart from this direct gene stimulation Vitamin D also affects the so-called epigenetics, conveying that certain genes can be switched on and off or even permanently off by methylation. Vitamin D must therefore be a genetic modulator." A study done in 2014 confirms this. (100)

Vitamin D receptors – docking stations

Research during the last decades established the initiation of diverse biological actions of 1,25-dihydroxycholecalciferol vitamin D3 through precise changes in gene expression. These are mediated by an intracellular vitamin D receptor.

In 2012 the "Sunshine vitamin D" study describes the activities of vitamin D receptor (VDR) as a binding protein. A receptor binds vitamin D on "genes and regulates the synthesis of numerous proteins, enzymes and neurotransmitters, which in turn control and influence numerous bodily processes." Research has found that the VDR significantly affects 229 genes, including genes that are associated with autoimmune conditions and cancer. (101)

Vitamin D receptors are found throughout the body on nearly every cell, from the sperm to the mitochondria. (102)

Here are some examples:
- eyes (103)
- pancreas (104)
- breast (89)
- fat-tissue
- brain (102)
- immune system (105)
- skin (106)
- bone (107)
- liver (108)
- muscle (109)
- parathyroid
- nervous system (110)
- kidney

- prostate (111)
- gastrointestinal tract (112)
- spermatozoon (113)
- DNA (114)
- and more

Ideal vitamin D-level as seen in blood serum

The Endocrine Society Clinical Practice Guidelines Committee gives recommendations to physicians for the treatment and prevention of vitamin D deficiency. "They encourage a level at least of 30 ng/ml. 40 to 60 ng/ml as a good range. Levels up to 100 ng/ml have been proven to be perfectly safe and healthy." (115)

Grassroots Health, a non-profit community service organization dedicated to promoting public awareness about vitamin D, has assembled a database that includes information on the supplemental vitamin D intake. They base their recommendations on several cohort studies. They link these intakes to the measured values for serum 25(OH)D, various demographic variables, and an array of health status measures. (116)

"Evaluation in adults suggests vitamin D levels less than approximately 30 ng/ml are considered vitamin D insufficient." (89)

Long term safety

In 2003 The *British Medical Journal* published a double-blind controlled test of 100,000 IU vitamin D3 given orally to over 2,000 elderly patients once every two months. The effects were monitored over a period of 5 years. The authors reported, in addition to greatly reduced fracture rates, that the high-dose therapy was "without adverse effects in men and women." (117)

Chart of Vitamin D levels vs disease - Grassroots Health June 2013 (118)

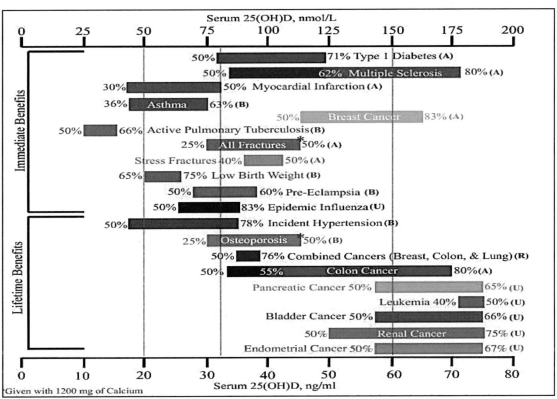

Source: www.grassrootshealth.net

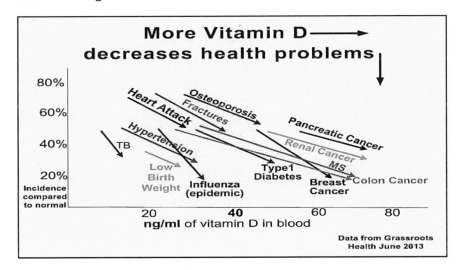

Source: www.grassrootshealth.net

Vitamin D in action

The following chapters will grant you some insight into the current medical mainstream research and the accumulation of scientific evidence proving that vitamin D has therapeutic benefits. The studies are executed with smaller or larger groups and give the conclusions of the researchers.

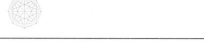

More in depth research is currently underway and continuously showing the value and importance of vitamin D.

We are born to live.
The immune system watches over life processes.
Support or destroy -
The immune system decides.

The Immune System and Vitamin D

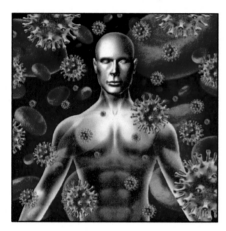

The immune system is the body's defense against infectious organisms and other invaders. Through a series of steps called the immune response, the immune system attacks organisms and substances that invade our systems and cause diseases. The immune system is made up of a network of cells, tissues, and organs working together to protect the body and its interaction with the environment.

The **innate immune** system, also known as the non-specific immune system or the in-born immune system, is an important subsystem of the overall immune system involving all the cells and mechanisms that defend the host from infection by other organisms.

The main components of the innate immune system:
- physical epithelial barriers
- phagocytic leukocytes
- dendritic cells
- a special type of lymphocyte called a natural killer (NK) cell
- circulating plasma proteins.

The **adaptive or acquired** immune system is composed of highly specialized, systemic cells and processes that eliminate a host of infectious agents, including bacteria, viruses, fungi, and parasites or prevent their excess growth. This process of acquired immunity is the basis of vaccination. (119)
The adaptive immune system develops in the course of each individual life and responds to personal experiences such as critical life events, feelings and actions.

There are two types of adaptive immune responses:
- humoral immunity, mediated by antibodies produced by B lymphocytes,
- cell-mediated immunity, mediated by T lymphocytes

Vitamin D is an essential protecting and lifesaving strategist for the immune system. Sufficient levels of Vitamin D reduce the risk of infectious disease by strengthening both immune systems. A 2011 study affirms that "vitamin D turns key peptides on in the immune system. This triggers a strong anti-microbial response, allowing the body to quickly and effectively repel invaders before they can develop into a full-blown infection." (120) Deficiency in vitamin D is associated with increased autoimmunity as well as an increased susceptibility to infection. (121)

Vitamin D and protective immunity

Vitamin D has been used to treat infections such as tuberculosis long before effective antibiotics were present. Physicians sent tuberculosis patients to sanatoriums. The treatment here included exposure to sunlight. The antiviral and antibacterial effect of vitamin D cured the tuberculosis. (121) Cod liver oil, a rich source of vitamin D, was in countless cases part of a treatment for tuberculosis as well as a nutritious diet. (122)

Pulmonary tuberculosis cured with sunlight

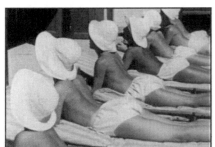

1914 St. Moritz (Switzerland): Boys with pulmonary tuberculosis sunbathing - after 12 months of sun exposure and oxygen-rich mountain air, the tuberculosis was healed. Sunbathing was at this time integral part treating tuberculosis. Hospitals were built with sunbathing facilities. Nurses wheeled the patient's bed directly out onto verandas, balconies, or decks for sunlight bathing. (123)

Physicians prescribed sun treatment to tuberculosis patients for several reasons. First of all, the sun acts as a bactericide, killing the tubercular bacillus organisms that cause the disease. One assumed that moderately hot temperatures sufficiently kill off these bacteria and clear up infections. Furthermore, ergosterol, present in the skin converts into vitamin D with the sun's UV rays. This was believed to do further damage to the TB bacilli. (124)

Bone tuberculosis cured with sunlight

In 1895 in Engadin, Switzerland Oscar Bernhard was the main initiator for establishing the highest altitude hospital of Europe in Samedan. Here he started his sunlight therapy. He discovered this idea by studying the dry meat preparation. The drying and the bactericidal effect of the sun contributed to the long shelf life of dried beef. (125)

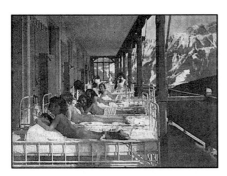

This principle also works in humans. After an initial successful attempt on an infected and poorly healing abdominal wound, Bernhard began treating patients with fistulas, tubercular ulcers and finally even bone tuberculosis with sunlight. He is generally regarded as the first heliotherapist of the modern era. In 1903, another Swiss physician, Dr. Auguste Rollier began to use sun baths at his tuberculosis clinic at Leysin, Switzerland. He became heliotherapy's most celebrated practitioner. (126)

Source: notresaga.com

There are many reports, that other doctors worldwide used the UV rays of sunlight to treat diseases such as tuberculosis, rickets, smallpox, lupus vulgaris and various other wounds. (127)

Andreas Moritz, in his book *Heal Yourself with Sunlight* states, "by the year 1933, there were over 165 diseases for which sunlight was proven to be a beneficial treatment. By the 1960's, manmade 'miracle drug antibiotics' replaced the fascination for the sun's healing power. By 1980 the public was increasingly bombarded with warnings about sunbathing and the risk of skin cancer." (127)

Genius T-cells – recognize and terminate

Lymphocytes are special immune cells. They recognize and remember invading bacteria and viruses. T-cells originate as undifferentiated white blood cells in the bone marrow. They travel through the blood system to the thymus, where they mature and are transformed into T-cells. These T-cells defend against viruses, bacteria, fungi and other diseases. T-cells are unusually effective at attacking antigen, or molecular sites, specific to acute and chronic lymphoblastic leukemia, and melanoma.

There are billions of different kinds of T-cells, each of them sufficiently trained to recognize one particular antigen. An antigen is a substance that can stimulate the production of antibodies and can connect specifically with them.

The identification of one special antigen by a single T-cell is one of the most outstanding aspects of the adaptive immune response. "The human immune system can recognize a staggering 100 billion different antigens displayed on the surface of the phagocytes." Based on that recognition, the adaptive immune system is able to "customize its terminator strategy" to each particular antigen. (128)

T-cells come in many categories with specific functions, including:
- Helper T-cells direct the immune system. Helper T-cells are also the cells attacked by the AIDS virus.
- Cytotoxic T-cells release certain chemicals that defile and kill invading organisms.
- Memory T-cells remain after this process to help the immune system respond more quickly once the same unfriendly organism is encountered again.
- Suppressor T-cells suppress the immune response so it does not destroy normal cells once the immune response has done its job.

Studies have shown a strong influence and dependency of vitamin D for proper T-cell function. (129) Researchers conclude in a study done in 2000 that "In principle, vitamin D exposure leads to a shift from a pro-inflammatory to a more tolerogenic immune status, including very diverse effects on T-cells." (130)

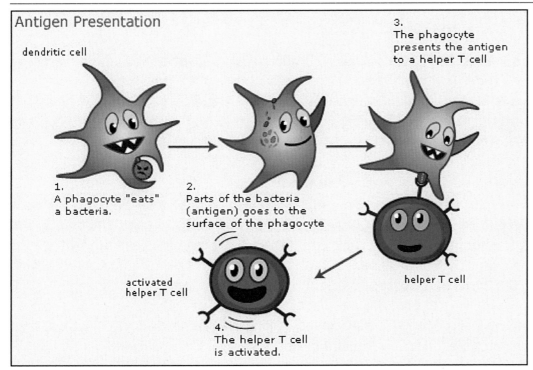

Antigen Presentation

dendritic cell

3.
The phagocyte presents the antigen to a helper T cell

1.
A phagocyte "eats" a bacteria.

2.
Parts of the bacteria (antigen) goes to the surface of the phagocyte

helper T cell

activated helper T cell

4.
The helper T cell is activated.

Source: www.nobelprize.org

Asthma attacks reduced with vitamin D

Asthma is a common chronic disease, affecting about 300 million people worldwide. The symptoms of asthma include wheezing, coughing, chest tightness, and shortness of breath. Vitamin D has several effects on the innate and adaptive immune systems:

- in the primary prevention of asthma.
- modulation of the severity of asthma exacerbations.
- reduction of asthma morbidity.

A new Cochrane Review published in the Cochrane Library (2016) has found evidence from randomized trials that "taking an oral vitamin D supplement in addition to standard asthma medication is likely to reduce severe asthma attacks." (131)

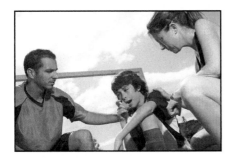 The team of Cochrane researchers conducted seven experiments involving 435 children and two studies, involving 658 adults. The participants were ethnically diverse, reflecting the broad range of global geographic settings, involving Canada, India, Japan, Poland, the UK, and the US. Most people continued to take their usual asthma medication while participating in the studies. The studies lasted between six and 12 months. (132)

The researchers found that giving an oral vitamin D supplement "reduced the risk of severe asthma attacks from 8 percent to around 3 percent." The Cochrane Review's lead author, Professor Adrian Martineau from the Asthma UK Centre for Applied Research, Queen Mary University of London, stated, "We found that taking a vitamin D supplement in addition to standard asthma treatment significantly reduced the risk of severe asthma attacks, without causing side effects." (133)

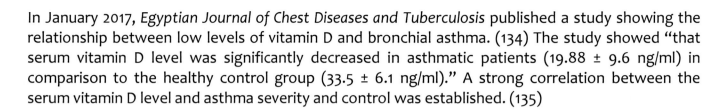

In January 2017, *Egyptian Journal of Chest Diseases and Tuberculosis* published a study showing the relationship between low levels of vitamin D and bronchial asthma. (134) The study showed "that serum vitamin D level was significantly decreased in asthmatic patients (19.88 ± 9.6 ng/ml) in comparison to the healthy control group (33.5 ± 6.1 ng/ml)." A strong correlation between the serum vitamin D level and asthma severity and control was established. (135)

Cutting influenza risk with vitamin D rather than vaccines
The annual flu season usually begins when the sun's intensity decreases. In the Northern hemisphere this is as early as end of August. During the flu season we have less light than in the spring and summer. If it is cold, people spend their time increasingly indoors. Less sunlight means less vitamin D. It is not the virus that causes the flu. It is the vitamin D deficiency that causes an acid environment and makes the body more susceptible to infection and disease.

A study (136) shows that 90 percent of the participants taking sufficient vitamin D were spared from the common flu. Thirty percent of the vitamin D deficient control group suffered a cold. (137)

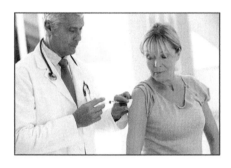

"Additional vitamin D intake effectively reduces the risk of an influenza infection better than vaccines or antiviral drugs," according to a study by scientists at the Medical Faculty of the Jikei University in Tokyo, which was published in the *American Journal of Clinical Nutrition*. (138) The Japanese researchers concluded "that the anti-viral drugs Zanamivir and Oseltamivir reduce risk of flu infection by 8 percent in children who have been exposed to infection, compared to a 50 percent or greater reduction with vitamin D." (139)

Studies, done in the United States and Germany come to the same conclusion. A better vitamin D status enhances response to vaccination and immunization. Sufficient vitamin D levels may improve protection of older people from influenza illness after flu immunization. (140)

Allergies and vitamin D

Vitamin deficiency is linked to food allergies
When it comes to food, the response of the immune system is naturally tolerant. Modern lifestyle food, chronic emotional and physical stress and food additives become a growing challenge for the immune response.

Food allergies are the consequence of over reactive immune responses to common and otherwise harmless food antigens.

- Food allergies are an abnormal immune reaction consisting of hypersensitivity to food components. The incidence of food allergies is increasing in children.

- Congruent with the increase of food allergies is an "epidemic of vitamin D deficiency caused by several factors, especially decreased sunlight/UVB exposure." These facts were established in a study published in 2010. (141)

Food allergies are five times more likely with low vitamin D (142)

In 2014 *ResearchGate* published a study. The objective of the study was to investigate *The Link between Serum Vitamin D Level, Sensitization to Food Allergens, and the Severity of Atopic Dermatitis in Infancy.* The results show that a "vitamin D deficiency increases the risk of sensitization to food allergens and that atopic dermatitis may be more severe in infants with vitamin D deficiency." (143)

Multiple food allergies appear ten times more likely with low vitamin D levels

Complete data was obtained from a total of 481 infants. Researchers concluded, that "in those classified as food sensitized (361), infants with vitamin D insufficiency were 3 times more likely to have food allergies than to be food-sensitized tolerant. For infants of Australian-born parents (271), vitamin D-insufficient infants were three times more likely to have any food allergy, ten times more likely to have multiple food allergies." (144)

The skin responds to vitamin D

The human skin is the outer covering of the body. It weighs about 2 to 3 kilograms and sheds itself about once every 27 days. It is the largest organ of the integumentary system. The integumentary system works to waterproof, cushion and protect the body from infection.

Wound healing and skin repair benefit from vitamin D

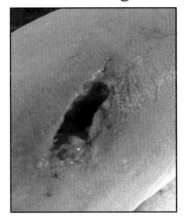

The skin provides the major barrier to all life threatening forces in the environment. Once this barrier is disrupted, the body loses fluids and is at risk of penetrating infectious organisms. It is essential that wound healing is efficient. The healing process should protect the body from both losses of essential fluids and infection.

Vitamin D and calcium play an important role in the healing of wounds. Vitamin D activates the cell to cell communication restoring and reconnecting of tissue. It also enhances stem cell production. Stem cells provide "keratinocytes not only for hair follicle formation but also for the reepithelization of the epidermis after wounding. The function of these bulge stem cells is regulated by vitamin D nuclear receptor. Vitamin D signaling is necessary for a normal innate immune response in the epidermis." (145)

Vitamin D regulates wound healing by
- enabling the initial inflammatory response of the epidermis to wounding.
- controlling the proliferation and migration of keratinocytes to close the wound.
- stimulating the differentiation of the keratinocytes to reform the permeability barrier through mechanisms requiring certain peptides. (146)

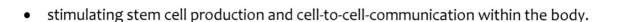

- stimulating stem cell production and cell-to-cell-communication within the body.

In 2014 the *National Institute of Health* published an article about *The role of vitamin D and calcium signaling in wound healing*. The author Daniel Bikle confirms the importance of vitamin D in wound healing, "vitamin D controls genes that promote the creation of cathelicidin. The immune system uses cathelicidin as an antimicrobial peptide to fight off wound infections. Calcium is as well a critical participant in the mechanism by which vitamin D signaling regulates these processes in keratinocytes. Calcium, like vitamin D, induces the genes responsible for differentiation, and limits proliferation." (147)

Acne responds to vitamin D
The skin has tiny holes called pores, which can get blocked by oil, bacteria, dead skin cells, and dirt. Acne, medically known as Acne Vulgaris, is a skin disease that involves the oil glands at the base of hair follicles. It commonly occurs during puberty when the sebaceous (oil) glands are activated. These are stimulated by male hormones produced by the adrenal glands of both males and females.

Since vitamin D functions as hormone, a deficiency creates an imbalance between other hormones in the body. This can disrupt the way the skin produces oily substances. This imbalance often results in acne.
- Vitamin D is known to stimulate T-cells to fight off infection in the skin.
- It suppresses sebaceous gland activity.
- It helps regulate the skin's sebum production.
- It decreases overactive cell turnover which keeps pores from getting clogged with dead skin cells.

In a study conducted as early as 1938, the beneficial effect of vitamin D on acne was proven. "Out of 70 patients, a skin improvement could be witnessed in 20 patients after three months, 32 of them were even healed. Many acne patients report that their skin appearance improved in the summer." (148)

Neurodermatitis benefits from vitamin D
Atopic dermatitis or eczema is a chronic inflammatory disease of the skin. It is uncomfortable and makes patients more susceptible to bacterial infections. The symptoms of the disease often worsen in the winter. (149)

Vitamin D deficiency plays a significant role in skin diseases, such as neurodermatitis (atopic eczema), psoriasis or vitiligo. A study involving 95 neurodermatitis patients revealed that patients with a lower level of vitamin D exhibited an increased frequency of bacterial skin infections. The results of a further study, which examined the effect of high doses of vitamin D on the clinical course of psoriasis und vitiligo, reported "positive results in the treatment of diseases with vitamin D in all 9 psoriasis patients and in 14 out of 16 vitiligo patients. These patients showed a re-pigmentation of 25-75 percent." (150)

A study done by Immunology and Allergy Clinics of North America (89) verifies, "Given the potential for vitamin D to suppress inflammatory responses, enhance antimicrobial peptide activity, and promote the integrity of the permeability barrier, supplementation provides a possible therapeutic intervention for a variety of skin disorders, including atopic dermatitis." (151)

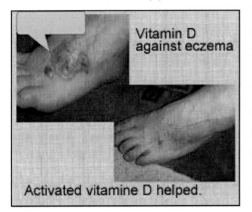

Vitamin D against eczema

Activated vitamine D helped.

Dr. Raymond von Helden, a general practitioner in Germany, diabetologist and vitamin D expert researched intensively and successfully with vitamin D. Here is a patient with eczema. This skin disease responded to none of the usual therapies. Even cortisone was of no avail. Only a treatment with active vitamin D initiated the healing process. (152)

Source: www.vitamindelta.de

In 2008 the Journal Allergy Clinical Immunology published a double-blind randomized controlled trial. The trial was performed with children suffering from winter-related atopic dermatitis. The children received 1,000 IU/day of vitamin D for one month during the winter. Five children received this aforementioned supplementation versus placebos for six children. "Baseline changes in the overall appearance of the skin showed that the vitamin D treatment group had a significant improvement in baseline score compared to placebo. (153)

Scleroderma and psoriasis benefit from vitamin D and UVB

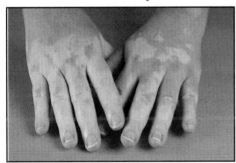

Scleroderma is a rheumatic disease and a connective tissue disease. It affects tissues such as skin, tendons, and cartilage. **Psoriasis** is a skin disease that causes scaly red patches of skin. Sometimes people with psoriasis develop joint pains, which are called psoriatic arthritis. **Leukoderma** – the skin whitening disease is a gradual loss of pigment melanin from the skin layers resulting in white patches on the surface of skin. **Vitiligo** is a specific kind of leukoderma.

Over many centuries, treatment with sunlight or heliotherapy was used in the therapy of skin diseases. More than 3,500 years ago, ancient Egyptian and Indian healers used sunlight for treating leucoderma.

With the discovery of ultraviolet radiation by Niels Ryberg Finsen all types of skin diseases were extensively treated with radiation. The radiation treatment not only disinfects and/or sterilizes various micro-organisms but also helps produce vitamin D3. Vitamin D in turn increases immunity in the human body. "Complete healings were reported in 80 percent of the cases." (154)

Scleroderma has responded favorably to long-term oral vitamin D3 therapy (155) and psoriasis has been successfully treated, not only with vitamin D supplements, but also with topical vitamin D3. (154)

Damage by radioactivity drastically reduced with vitamin D

In 2003 a study of the Bundeswehr (German armed forces) proved that skin cells were protected by vitamin D hormones from the damage by ionizing radiation.

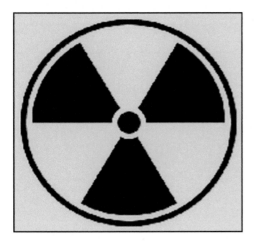

This was confirmed in 2005 by a study in Turkey on the skin cells of rats. The rats received a dose of harmful radiation as used for children with leukemia: 20 Gray. With the mere administration of only 0.2 micrograms of vitamin D, the resulting 8 IU of vitamin D3 caused a significant protection of the hair follicles.

In 2010 the Saarland group of Prof W. Tilgen and Jörg Reichrath of the University Homburg / Saar confirmed in a cell experiment the protection of the skin cells by vitamin D. Calcitriol, which protects the skin cells against damage caused by ionizing radiation. (156)

During the atomic bomb tests in the South Pacific (Bikini Atoll) the people living there were more exposed to radiation than the observant soldiers on the ships, who originated from the US and UK. Subsequent illnesses such as Leukemia were found mainly in the soldiers, while the people of the South Seas were rarely suffering from this type of cancer. (157)

Vitamin D may improve survival in a mustard gas attack

Sulfur Mustard is a potent alkylating agent with electrophilic property which has been used as a chemical warfare agent most recently by ISIS. (158) A study published in 2016 specifies the skin damage after mustard gas attacks. "If not inhaled, mustard gas kills by eroding the skin and attacking underlying muscles and the internal organs. It literally eats through the skin and muscle like an acid that cannot be washed away. Mustard gas has been used by about 10 countries in different wars. To date, there is no effective treatment for mustard gas."

In April of 2016, researchers at Case Western Reserve University validated the first treatment for mustard gas: Vitamin D. "The mortality rate when using vitamin D significantly decreases." (159)

We are born to live.
The nervous system governs and controls life processes.
Fight or flight – this is one of the questions.

The Nervous System and Vitamin D

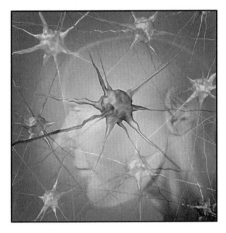

The nervous system is a highly specialized network system that contains countless neurons. They receive, process and transmit signals between different parts of the body. The nervous system allows us to perceive, comprehend, and respond to the world around us.

The nervous system has two major parts
- the central nervous system.
- and the peripheral nervous system.

The central nervous system consists of the brain and spinal cord. It is responsible for sending, receiving and interpreting information from all parts of the body.

The peripheral nervous system consists of a network of nerves that connects the body to the central nervous system. It serves as a communication relay between the brain and other parts of the body. The peripheral nervous system functions through two separate yet intricately connected systems:

The autonomic nervous system
It influences the function of internal organs. This control system governs life processes and regulates bodily functions such as the heart rate, digestion, respiratory rate, pupillary response, urination, and sexual arousal. This system is the primary mechanism in control of the fight-or-flight response and the freeze-and-dissociate response.

The somatic system
It consists of nerves that connect the brain and spinal cord with muscles and sensory receptors in the skin. It involves parts of the body a person can command at will. It regulates the functions that serve the active, individual relationship with the outside world, including own thought processes and nutrition.

The nervous system can suffer from a number of afflictions:
- Multiple sclerosis (MS) is characterized by destruction of the myelin sheath that insulates and protects neurons.
- Meningitis causes an inflammation of the membranes surrounding the brain and spinal cord.
- Alzheimer's disease.
- Parkinson's disease.
- Epilepsy.
- Shingles.

- Stroke.
- many forms of cancer.
- mental attitudes and environmental influences.

A team of researchers led by Dr. Guang-Xian Zhang and colleagues published a new study in Experimental and *Molecular Pathology* investigating *The role of vitamin D in promoting neural repair by stimulating the growth and maturation of neural stem cells*. "Overall, we demonstrated that 1,25(OH)2D3 has a direct effect on the neural stem cell proliferation, survival, and neuron/oligodendrocyte differentiation. This represents a novel mechanism underlying its remyelinating and neuroprotective effect in MS and encephalomyelitis therapy." (160)

Connection between vitamin D and the nervous system including the brain

Vitamin D has neuroprotective and immunomodulatory effects on the brain and nervous system. It belongs to the group of neurosteroids - a group of hormones that have direct effect on function and development of nerve cells, neurons and the brain. (161)

A study published in Trends in *endocrinology and metabolism* about *New clues about vitamin D functions in the nervous system* reports of the discovery of "nuclear receptors for 1,25(OH)(2)D(3) in neurons and glial cells. Genes encoding the enzymes involved in the metabolism of this hormone are also expressed in brain cells." (162)

The reported biological effects of vitamin D
- prevent oxidative damage to nervous tissue and increases glutathione levels.
- help detoxify pathways and maintain correct formation and maintenance of neuronal connections.
- control the cell cycle of nerve cells and the neuroplasticity.
- influence the synthesis of neurotransmitters, supports cell-to-cell-communication.
- control the formation of important antioxidants and affects the detoxification of the brain.
- regulate the expression of over 200 genes. (163)
- support intracellular calcium homeostasis.
- activate remyelination.

Depression responds to vitamin D

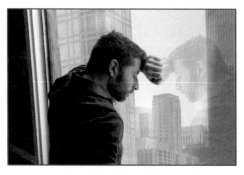

Depression has many possible causes, including faulty mood regulation by the brain, genetic vulnerability, stressful life events, medications, and medical problems.

Depression is one of the leading causes of disability in the United States. It is a known risk factor. It affects 350 million people worldwide. It is the leading cause of disability and the fourth-leading cause of the global disease burden. The statistical risk of suffering from depression has almost doubled in young adults, according to a recent study. (164)

Connection between vitamin D and depression

The association between depressive disorders and vitamin D deficiency from a lack of sun exposure is well established and was first noted two thousand years ago. (165) Depressed people often have extremely low vitamin D levels. (166)

Researchers at the Department of Psychiatry and Behavioral Neuroscience at St. Joseph's Hospital in Hamilton, Ontario Province, Canada revealed a connection between vitamin D levels and depression. (167) It is known that vitamin D receptors are present in the brain. Enzymes involved in vitamin D hydroxylation are present throughout the central nervous system.

Epidemiological evidence shows that "Vitamin D deficiency is associated with an 8–14 percent increase in depression" (168) and a 50 percent increase in suicide. "Causality and efficacy of supplementation remain controversial awaiting confirmation by systematic review and meta-analysis." (169)
A meta-analysis of various available studies from 2013 up to 2016 concluded "the greater the Vitamin D deficiency is, the worse the symptoms of depression are. An increase of the vitamin D levels in turn leads to a degeneration of the symptom." (167)

Depression in wintertime

Not the cold weather makes us sad and heat that makes us happy. It is the missing of the sun's uplifting qualities. Too little light may trigger depression; but too much light may trigger mania in some people. People with maniac depression are especially sensitive to light and thus more likely to have seasonal mood swings. In fact, in the first modern studies of seasonal affective disorder (SAD) in the 1980s, winter depression was accompanied by spring hypomania in 92 percent of subjects. In other words SAD was the same illness as seasonality in bipolar disorder. (170)

Bipolar disorder and vitamin D

Bipolar disorder is a psychiatric condition in which an individual transitions between spells of depression and mania. Approximately 5.7 million adults in the United States are affected with this condition. The vitamin D status has been linked to neuropsychiatric illness, including but not limited to depression status, seasonal affective disorder and schizophrenia.

A recent study published by the *Journal of Clinical Psychopharmacology* found individuals "who have bipolar disorder were 4.7 times more likely to be vitamin D deficient. Of the 118 participants with bipolar disorder 20.3 percent had optimal levels, 25.4 percent were sufficient, 31.4 percent were insufficient and 22.9 percent were vitamin D deficient."

The researchers concluded, "In this study vitamin D deficiency was found to be 4.7 times more common in a population of 320 outpatients with bipolar disorder, schizophrenia, or schizoaffective disorder." (171)

Pregnancy and mood disorders

Mood disorders in pregnancy and post-partum period are common. Researchers have studied the relationship between low serum vitamin D concentration and perinatal depression. The randomized clinical trial was tested on pregnant women who were under prenatal care in a teaching hospital in Shiraz, Iran. The study published in 2016 showed that "consuming 2,000 IU vitamin D3 daily during late pregnancy was effective in decreasing perinatal depression levels." (172)

Parkinson's disease responds to vitamin D

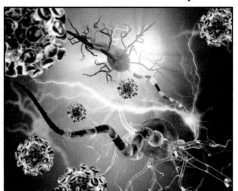

Parkinson's disease is a neurodegenerative disorder associated with a loss of nerve cells that produce dopamine. Tremors, slow movement, muscle rigidity and difficulty walking are experienced. Additionally, many patients are plagued with a variety of secondary complications from the disease. (173) It is recognized as the second most common neurodegenerative disorder after Alzheimer's disease. Parkinson's disease has a great impact on the quality of life. It significantly affects the ability to carry out daily activities due to both motor and non-motor symptoms and complications of medical treatment.

(174)

The Connection between Vitamin D and Parkinson's disease

Scientists have discovered that vitamin D receptors are most strongly expressed in dopamine-rich regions of the brain. Researchers believe that this may explain the neuroprotective role of vitamin D in several brain disorders, including Parkinson's. (175) Vitamin D may have both protective and symptomatic effects in Parkinson's disease. The scientists in a study published 2016 concluded "that vitamin D plays a neuroprotective and neurotrophic role in the brain." (176)

Vitamin D council published an article on *New trial says vitamin D prevents progression and deterioration of Parkinson's Disease.* The author writes about the very low vitamin D-levels seen in Parkinson's patients compared to their healthy counterparts. "Additionally, vitamin D has been proven to prevent the progression and deterioration of Parkinson's disease." (177)

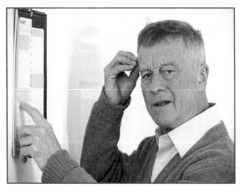

Dementia and vitamin D

Dementia is a general term for the decline in mental ability severe enough to interfere with daily life. Dementia may include memory loss and difficulties with thinking, problem-solving or language. A person with dementia may also experience changes in their mood or behavior.

One cause of dementia is when the brain is damaged by diseases such as Alzheimer's disease. Dementia has different causes too. Heavy metal intoxication is one of them. The specific symptoms that someone with dementia experiences will depend on the parts of the brain that are damaged and the disease that is causing the dementia. (178) Dementia has been diagnosed in people in their 50's, 40's and even in their 30's. Juvenile dementia (age 8 and up) is on the rise in the U.S. due to mothers eating a no-fat diet. (179)

The Connection between Vitamin D and Dementia

An international research team conducted a study that monitored over 1,600 seniors for six years. They found "that those who were severely deficient in vitamin D were more than twice more likely to develop Alzheimer's and dementia than those who had adequate levels. Participants who were only mildly deficient had an increased risk of 53 percent, while those who were severely deficient had a 125 percent increased risk of developing dementia." (180)

Lead author David Llewellyn of the University of Exeter Medical School said, "We expected to find an association between low vitamin D levels and the risk of dementia and Alzheimer's disease, but the results were surprising – we actually found that the association was twice as strong as we anticipated." (181)

Some 44 million people worldwide have dementia, a number that is expected to triple by 2050. On the other hand researchers assume, that about one billion people around the globe vitamin D deficient. (181)

Autism responds to vitamin D

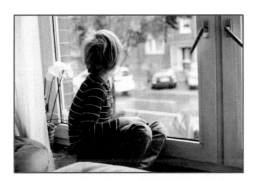

Autism describes a range of conditions categorized as neurodevelopmental disorders. Characteristics of autism include deficits in social skills, impairment in verbal and nonverbal communication and repetitive patterns of behavior, interests or activities. Individuals with mild autism may have exceptional intellectual abilities. It affects how a person communicates with and relates to other people, and how they experience the world around them.

The Centers for Disease Control and Prevention reported in 2010 that one in every 110 children born in 2002 was diagnosed with autism by age 8. In 2012, statistics have shown that one out of every 68 eight-year-olds in the US has been diagnosed with autism. (182)

The connection between vitamin D and autism

Vitamin D plays an essential role in neurodevelopment and gene regulation. More than 2,700 genes contain vitamin D receptors, and vitamin D regulates the expression of over 200 genes. Furthermore, vitamin D deficiency during pregnancy is associated with adverse effects for the baby, including an increased risk of autism. (183) According to several studies, more children with autism are born during the spring, which is the time of year with the lowest vitamin D levels in northern latitudes.

A random controlled study was performed on 109 children ages three to ten years. All the children were diagnosed with autism. Half of the children were randomly chosen to receive a daily vitamin D

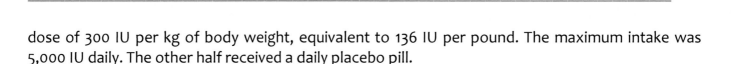

dose of 300 IU per kg of body weight, equivalent to 136 IU per pound. The maximum intake was 5,000 IU daily. The other half received a daily placebo pill.

After four months of vitamin D supplementation parents and occupational therapists reported significantly improved participation in social life, more concentration, less irritability, stereotypic behavior or inappropriate speech. The parents and therapists of placebo group children did not experience any significant improvements.

The study researchers conclude, "Children who received vitamin D supplementation experienced increased cognitive awareness, social awareness and social cognition compared to those who only received the placebo. Vitamin D supplementation significantly decreased repetitive hand movements, random noises, jumping and restricted interests." (184)

Epilepsy seizures respond to vitamin D

Epilepsy is a chronic brain disorder that affects more than 55 million people worldwide. (185) Epileptic seizures result from abnormal electrical activity in the brain. They can strike at any age and time and are distinct by various signs. Several types of seizure with open eyes are experienced or impairment of consciousness with a blank stare. This depends on the brain region, which is affected. Epilepsy is the fourth most common neurological disorder and affects people of all ages.

The connection between vitamin D and epilepsy

Vitamin D is a fat soluble steroid. Researchers followed the thread of causes and treatments of epilepsy. A vitamin deficiency has been seen in all cases of epilepsy. (186) Researchers review "evidence supporting a link between vitamin D and epilepsy including those coming from ecological as well as interventional and animal studies. Converging evidence indicates a role for vitamin D deficiency in the pathophysiology of epilepsy." (187)

A pilot study done in 2012 concludes, "We found that seizure numbers significantly decreased with vitamin D3 supplementation. The average seizure reduction was 40 percent. We conclude that the normalization of serum vitamin 25(OH)D level has an anticonvulsant effect." (188)

Multiple Sclerosis responds to vitamin D

Multiple Sclerosis (MS) is a disease of autoimmunity and inflammation characterized by the destruction of the myelin sheath. This special very sensitive sheath insulates and protects neurons. The immune system attacks the central nervous system with impact on the brain, spinal cord and optic nerves. The symptoms come and go in the beginning. Strange sensations, fatigue, heat-related or walking problems are some of the first indications. Once MS is manifest, "attacks" or phases of increased disease activity are experienced.

Medical News Today published in 2015 a study "that daily sun exposure during adolescence and a lower body mass index may delay the development of multiple sclerosis." (189)

The connection between vitamin D and MS

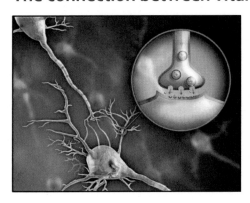

Vitamin D governs remyelination. Myelin sheaths are generated around axons in the adult central nervous system. The body has the innate ability to remyelinate nerve fibers and to repair any damage. This ability declines over time as the MS process continually attacks myelin.

A study conducted at Maastricht University in the Netherlands suggests that for people "who already have MS, vitamin D may lessen the frequency, progression and severity of their symptoms." (190)

Oligodendrocytes are the specialized cells that create the myelin sheath. These cells, in turn, are formed from precursor cells called oligodendrocyte progenitor cells. (191) A cascade of interaction between protein and receptors follows. A linking protein for the cascade of interactions between protein and receptors is the receptor binding vitamin D. The findings were published in The Journal of Cell Biology. (192)

The revelations of a study published 2015 in *Journal of Neurology* came to no surprise. Researchers report, "Low serum 25-hydroxyvitamin D (25[OH]D) levels are associated with an increased risk of MS as well as with increased disease activity and rate of progression in clinically isolated syndromes and early MS." The study included 1,482 patients from 26 countries. All these patients were treated with interferon beta-1b. Interferon beta-1b are small signaling proteins which help reduce the frequency in flare ups in MS patients. "In patients with MS treated with interferon beta-1b, higher 25(OH)D levels were associated with a lower rates of MS activity observed on MRI." (193)

The authors concluded, "The conclusions of this large prospective investigation consisting of patients from 5 continents and a broad range of serum 25(OH)D levels suggest that adequate vitamin D levels are an important determinant of MS activity not only during the disease development but also several years after the diagnosis. These results also suggest that individuals with MS may benefit from vitamin D levels above those currently considered by many to be sufficient in healthy adults." (194)

Vitamin D stimulating neural stem cells to reconstruction

A study done in 2015 demonstrated "vitamin D can stimulate neural stem cells into transforming into both myelin-producing oligodendrocytes and new nerve cells." (195) The following study went several steps further by showing that "stimulating these cells with vitamin D can repair myelin in animals with an MS-like disease. It also discovered the precise mechanisms by which vitamin D carries out its remyelinating actions." (196)

This study adds to a growing accumulation of scientific evidence showing that vitamin D might have potential therapeutic benefits beyond influencing the risk of developing MS. As the authors state, "further investigation into the molecular mechanisms of vitamin D receptors in remyelination will open up new opportunities for the development of regenerative medicines for demyelinating diseases. Specifically, these findings will help to create the design and interpretation of clinical tests studying the safety and effectiveness of vitamin D supplementation for treating the symptoms and/or disease development of MS, as earlier smaller scale trials have led to mixed results." (196)

Gray matter volume increase under vitamin D

A study discovered that "vitamin D status is positively associated with gray matter volume in patients with multiple sclerosis. Gray matter is responsible for processing information in the brain.

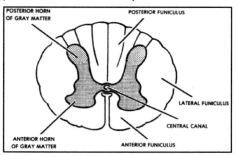

It is a known fact, that reductions in gray matter volume reflect neurodegeneration and disability in patients with MS." (197)

The researchers of a study published in 2016 confirmed "of the 65 patients, each 25 nmol/l (10 ng/ml) increase in 25(OH)D was associated with a 7.8 ml rise in grey matter volume (p = 0.025). Low vitamin D status was associated with a 44 percent increase of new brain lesions and a relapse within a year." (198)

Source: httpwww.indiana.edu

Multiple Sclerosis and geographic distribution

There is a very specific geographic distribution of this disease around the world. A significantly higher incidence of the disease is found in the northernmost latitudes and the southernmost latitudes. This observation is based on the incidence of the disease in Scandinavia, northern United States and Canada, as well as Australia and New Zealand. (199)

The link between vitamin D and MS is strengthened by the association between sunlight and the risk of MS. The farther away from the equator a person lives, the higher the risk of MS. Sunlight is the body's most efficient source for vitamin D — suggesting that exposure to sunlight may offer protection from MS. (200)

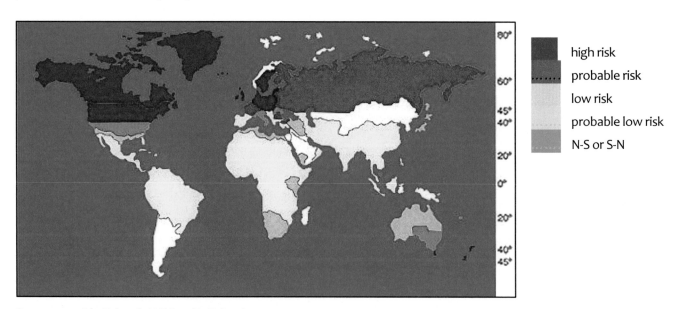

Source: 2008/9 Schools Wikipedia Selection

All blood vessels together in the human body encircle the globe three times.
Capillaries are often narrower than the red blood cells pressing through.
Could biophotons be the source for vascular drive?
Propelling cells thru capillaries.

Cardiovascular Disease and Vitamin D

Cardiovascular disease includes all the diseases of the heart and circulation including coronary heart disease, angina, heart attack, congenital heart disease and stroke. It is a major cause of morbidity and mortality worldwide. (201)

The connection between vitamin D and cardiovascular disease

Considerable evidence indicates that vitamin D
- is associated with cardiovascular disease risk factors. (202)
- is involved in the regulation of blood pressure, hypertension. (203)
- acts against chronic inflammation. (204)
- protects vessels and cardiac muscle directly. (205)

Low vitamin D levels can explain alterations in mineral metabolism as well as myocardial dysfunction in the congestive heart failure patients. It may be a contributing factor in the pathogenesis of congestive heart failure. (206) Not surprisingly, bone loss is associated with congestive heart failure. (207)

Hypertension lowered with vitamin D

Low 25(OH)D levels are an independent risk factor for prevalent and incident hypertension. (208) Meta-analyses of randomized controlled studies documented "that vitamin D supplementation lowers systolic blood pressure by 2–6 mmHg." (209) There are many publications available on the effect of vitamin D supplementation by cardiovascular disease. (210)

Mortality risk decreased with vitamin D

Beyond cardiovascular disease, vitamin D deficiency is associated with increased risk of total mortality. A meta-analysis with 6,853 patients suffering from cardiovascular disease "showed that mortality risk decreases by 14 percent by boosting 25(OH)D levels per 25 nm." (211) This recommendation corresponds to results of a meta-analysis including studies on frail, elderly patients. In this report vitamin D supplementation was associated with "a significant 7 percent decrease in total mortality." (212)

Another meta-analysis on vitamin D and its analogues reported a "significant mortality reduction in patients with the combined treatment of vitamin D plus calcium." (213) This study answers many worries about vitamin D intake and calcification. The researchers take a special effort to note "the

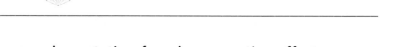

largest study on vitamin D plus calcium supplementation found no negative effect on coronary artery calcification." (214)

Parathyroid hormone suppressed with vitamin D

Epidemiological studies demonstrated that elevated and high-normal parathyroid hormone (PTH) levels are associated with an increased risk of cardiovascular events and mortality. (215) Clinical evidence on the effect of vitamin D status on cardiovascular risk factors proves that "PTH levels are inversely correlated with 25(OH) D concentrations." Researchers conclude in this study done in 2011 by scientists around Stefan Pilz at Division of Endocrinology and Metabolism, Department of Internal Medicine, Medical University of Graz, Austria, "PTH suppression by vitamin D supplementation might therefore reduce cardiovascular risk." (210)

Atherosclerosis effected – inflammation reduced

Clinical Endocrinology (210)

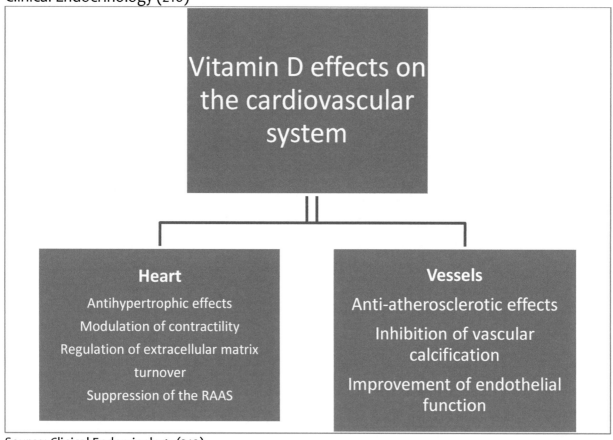

Source: Clinical Endocrinology (210)

Coronary heart disease (angina and heart attack) and stroke may be caused by the same dilemma called atherosclerosis. This is when arteries become narrow by a gradual build-up of fatty material, called atheroma, within their walls. It is the most common cause of heart disease. Previous research shows "that vitamin D may prevent atherosclerosis by reducing inflammation and arterial stiffness." (216)

Astounding metabolism!
10 million cells die every second
10 million cells are generated every second
Every second of your life!

Metabolism and Vitamin D

The metabolism is a complex system regulating all chemical reactions involved in maintaining the living state of the cells and the organism.

Metabolism can be divided into two categories:

- Catabolism involves all of the metabolic processes that obliterate biomolecules.
- Anabolism is all of the metabolic processes that build biomolecules.

Energy formation is one of the vital components of metabolism. Nutrition is the key. The pathways of metabolism rely on nutrients that they break down in order to produce biophotons or energy. (17) This energy in turn is required by the body to synthesize new proteins, nucleic acids (DNA, RNA), etc. (217)

Metabolic disorders occur when the metabolism process fails and causes the body to have either too much or too little of the essential substances needed to stay healthy. Metabolic disorders can appear in many forms. For instance:

- An enzyme or vitamin is missing, necessary for an important chemical reaction.
- Abnormal chemical reactions that hinder metabolic processes.
- Disease in the liver, pancreas, endocrine glands or other organs involved in metabolism.
- Nutritional deficiencies slow cell-regeneration down.

Bone health depends on calcium and vitamin D

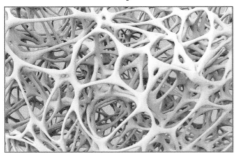

Bone is living tissue that is constantly being built up and down. The lifespan of bone cells is between 15 and 35 years. Metabolic bone diseases are disorders of bone strength. They are usually caused by abnormalities of minerals, such as calcium or phosphorus, vitamins, bone mass or bone structure. Osteoporosis, arthritis, rickets, bone cancer, osteomalacia, acromegaly, are just a few of the bone related disorders.

Rickets heals under sun exposure and vitamin D

Rickets affect the development of bones in children. It causes soft weak bones, which can become bowed or curved. It is a condition that only develops in children. It's most commonly diagnosed in children between the age of 3 and 18 months. The main signs and symptoms of rickets include a mis-shaped or deformed skeleton, pain, fragile bones, poor growth and development. The most common cause of rickets is an extreme lack of sunlight, vitamin D or a lack of calcium, or all of the above.

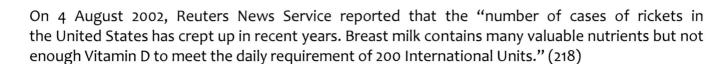

On 4 August 2002, Reuters News Service reported that the "number of cases of rickets in the United States has crept up in recent years. Breast milk contains many valuable nutrients but not enough Vitamin D to meet the daily requirement of 200 International Units." (218)

Adults can also develop soft and weak bones. This condition is called osteomalacia.

Osteoporosis responds to vitamin D

The body metabolizes and regenerates constantly bone cells. Osteoporosis occurs when more bone cells decay than new ones correctly generated. It causes bones to become weak and brittle – so brittle that a fall or even mild stress such as bending over or coughing can cause a fracture. Osteoporosis-related fractures most commonly develop in the hip, wrist or spine.

The study remarks, that "osteoporosis affects men and women of all races. White and Asian women – especially older women who are past menopause – are at highest risk." (219)

The connection between vitamin D and bone disorder

Vitamin D is essential for the development and maintenance of bone, both for its role in assisting calcium absorption from food in the intestine, and for ensuring the correct renewal and mineralization of bone tissue. (220)

Vitamin D
- is essential for ensuring the correct renewal and mineralization of bone tissue.
- controls the phosphate and calcium levels indirectly in the blood.
- ensures a constant blood calcium level with the parathyroid hormone.
- is responsible for the synthesis of two calcium-transporting proteins, osteocalcin and matrix GLA protein. These proteins provide calcium transport to bones and other places of activity and are needed for proper bone formation.

Most persons with osteoporosis have low vitamin D levels. Along with calcium, already a low dose of 800 IU vitamin D daily has been shown in a double-blind placebo-controlled study to "increase bone density, and to reduce hip fractures by an astounding 43 percent." (221) Vitamin D supplementation may decrease bone turnover and increase bone mineral density. Several randomized placebo-controlled trials with vitamin D and calcium showed a significant decrease in fracture occurrence. (222) Vitamin D and calcium for bone health require vitamin K2 to be activated. (223)

Less stress fractures under higher vitamin D levels

US researchers recommend that especially athletes and the elderly take a supplementation with vitamin D. "We recommend a serum vitamin D concentration of at least 40 ng/ml to active people with middle or higher functional demands, in order to prevent fatigue fractures," state the authors Dr. Jason R. Miller, foot and joint surgeon at the Pennsylvania Orthopedic Center in Malvern,

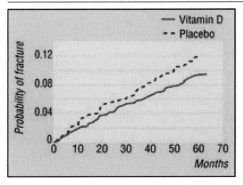

Source: BMJ volume 326, 1 March 2003

Pennsylvania, USA. "For effective fall and fracture prevention, an optimal threshold of at least 40 ng/ml is demanded by experts or professional associations. For these experts levels of 21 ng/ml vitamin D3 are considered insufficient." (224)

Periodontitis benefits from vitamin D

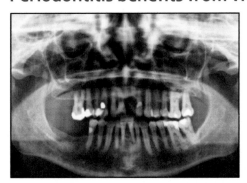

Periodontal disease is a chronic gum condition. Bacteria cause the gums to swell, redden, and bleed. Jaw bone tissue might become damaged. Periodontitis is defined as chronic bacterial infection that attacks the soft and bony hard tissue ultimately leading to tooth loss. Thus it was found in longitudinal studies that "low vitamin D levels in the body are associated with an increased rate of gingival inflammation and the loss of periodontal tissue." (225) The risk of periodontal disease increases with age.

The connection between sun-exposure, vitamin D, and periodontitis

A new study published in the *Journal of Clinical and Diagnostic Research* found that calcium and vitamin D supplementation improved markers against periodontitis. "According to our study, we received superior results on periodontal parameters by oral supplementation of low doses of calcium and vitamin D." (226)

A few studies indicate a direct role of sunlight in reducing the risk of periodontal disease.

- A study in Norway found "a direct relationship between tooth loss and latitude. Only 11 percent of people living in the south lost teeth compared to 43 percent living in the central region and 66 percent in the northern region. Ultraviolet B (UVB) light and vitamin D production decrease rapidly at higher latitudes."
- A study in Brazil found that "people with dark skin had a 50 to 60 percent greater risk of periodontitis than people with light skin." (227)

Obese people benefit from vitamin D

Obesity is a condition where a person has accumulated so much body fat that it might have a negative effect on their health. With a Body Mass Index (BMI) of 32 and more a person is considered obese, BMI between 26 and 31 the person is considered overweight. Obesity is determined by the following factors: genetics, behavior, environment, internally set points of weight, eating habits, and deficiency on vitamins and minerals.

Obesity is a health concern. Without proper treatment, obesity can lead to other serious health problems, such as:

- Osteoarthritis.
- heart disease and blood lipid abnormalities.
- stroke, type 2 diabetes, gallstones.
- sleep apnea (when you periodically stop breathing during sleep).
- reproductive problems.
- certain cancers.
- obesity hypoventilation syndrome.
- metabolic Syndrome.

The connection between vitamin D and obesity

A study published 2014 about the Importance of body weight for the dose relationship of oral vitamin D supplementation showed the relationship between obesity, BMI and vitamin D requirement. (228) Vitamin D deficiency is highly prevalent in overweight and obese persons. It is particularly highly prevalent in severely obese and minority children.

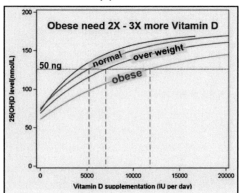

The *Clinical Practice Guidelines* by the Endocrine Society acknowledged "body weight differentials and recommend obese persons be given two to three times more vitamin D. This is due to decreased bioavailability of vitamin D in obesity." (229)

Source: www.vitaminwiki.com/tiki-index

Even more vitamin D is required

- by people with dark skin color.
- when consuming excess toxins such as DDT, PCB, alcohol, nicotine.
- by persons with health problems which require higher Vitamin D levels.
- for health problems which reduce the response of Vitamin D intake, especially problems of the liver (even fatty liver), kidney and colon.
- deficiency of cofactors such as magnesium, vitamin K2 and Omega-3.
- by smokers – known to reduce dose/response by 20 percent.
- after recent surgery/trauma – which consumes a lot of vitamin D.
- by persons taking drugs which reduce vitamin D levels - statins, chemotherapy, etc.
- by seniors, and
- by pregnant women.

Less weight gain with vitamin D

A study done in 2012 suggests the weight gain occurs in middle-aged women if vitamin D levels are lower than 30 ng. (230) The conclusions showed "higher 25(OH)D levels are associated with lower weight gains, suggesting low vitamin D status may predispose to fat accumulation." A study done January 2014 even suggests that vitamin D may block the obesity gene. (231)

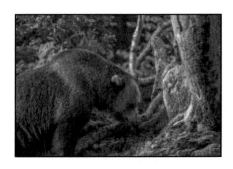

Right when the suns' intensity weakens, the brown bear prepares for hibernation. Grizzly bears gain 100-plus pounds prior to hibernation. Yet, unlike humans their cells do not stop responding to insulin and they do not develop type 2 diabetes or other metabolic diseases. Research shows that the bears' fat cells actually change their response to insulin depending on the season. They're sensitive to insulin in summertime, when the sun is at its highest. During preparation for hibernation they become insulin resistant. This resistance helps them gain the fat they need to survive the winter. When spring comes the vitamin D level rises, a normal metabolism sets in and the bears enjoy the summer in an active body.

Jeff Bowles, who experimented with extreme high doses vitamin D claims that the human metabolism functions under vitamin D deficiency similar to the brown bears metabolism shortly before hibernation. (232)

Diabetes and vitamin D

Diabetes is the most common metabolic disease. According to 2012 data from the American Diabetes Association, 29.1 million children and adults, or about 9.3 percent of the U.S. population has diabetes – with prevalence in seniors. (233) In general, people with diabetes either have a total lack of insulin (type 1 diabetes), have too little insulin or cannot use insulin effectively (type 2 diabetes).

Type 1 diabetes is when the body's immune system destroys the cells that release insulin, eventually eliminating the insulin production from the body. Without insulin, cells cannot absorb sugar (glucose). Yet glucose is crucial for the brain, for the energy metabolism and cell to cell communication. Over time, a lack of insulin can cause nerve and kidney damage, eyesight impairment, and increased risk of heart and vascular disease. The worldwide incidence rate of type 1 diabetes is steadily increasing. Approximately 1.25 million American children and adults have type 1 diabetes. Accumulating data shows that it is correlated with insufficient vitamin D.

Type 2 diabetes can develop at any age. It most commonly becomes apparent during adulthood. Type 2 diabetes in children is increasing. In type 2 diabetes, the body isn't able to use insulin effectively. This is called insulin resistance. As type 2 diabetes worsens, the pancreas produces less and less insulin. This is called insulin deficiency.

The body reacts to malnutrition, genetic disposition, and environmental factors in type 2 diabetes:
* the pancreas does not produce enough insulin to manage incoming glucose or
* the body becomes resistant to insulin.

When glucose starts to build up in the blood stream instead of being used or stored, it can cause diabetic complications. Complications include eyesight issues, skin conditions, diabetic feet and high blood pressure.

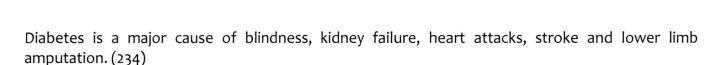

Diabetes is a major cause of blindness, kidney failure, heart attacks, stroke and lower limb amputation. (234)

The connection between vitamin D and diabetes

There is a wealth of evidence showing that vitamin D is necessary for insulin secretion. It reduces abnormal increases in insulin resistance in humans as well. (235)

- Vitamin D activates 1α-hydroxylase enzyme in the pancreas. (236)
- Vitamin D increases insulin sensitivity through the effect on its muscle cell receptors. (237)
- It controls blood glucose levels in type 1 diabetes. (238)
- Vitamin D protects against irreversible defects in islet cells, insulin resistance and related defects. (236)

According to recent research, vitamin D deficiency affects the glucose metabolism and may actually be more closely linked to diabetes than obesity. In a study done in 2016 with 118 people, "those with low vitamin D levels more likely to have type 2 diabetes, pre-diabetes or metabolic syndrome, regardless of their weight." (239)

A study published 2015 suggests "vitamin D deficiency and obesity interact synergistically to heighten the risk of diabetes and other metabolic disorders. The average person may be able to reduce their risk by maintaining a healthy diet and doing more outdoor activities." (240)

Another study published in 2013 found "that type 2 diabetics given 50,000 IUs of oral vitamin D3 per week for eight weeks experienced a meaningful reduction" in fasting plasma glucose and insulin. (241)

Experts say the prevalence of young diabetics has increased four-fold over a 20-year period, largely due to an increase in early onset of type 2 diabetes and less sun-exposure. (242)

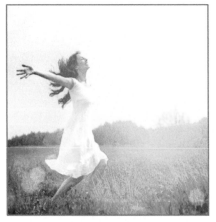

A study of more than 10,000 Finnish children who were given 2,000 IU vitamin D3 per day during the first year of life demonstrated a 78 percent reduced risk of type 1 diabetes over a 30-year follow-up. Subsequently, this finding was confirmed by a meta-analysis of five observational studies in England. (243)

Vitamin D deficiency has been associated with type 1 and type 2 diabetes as well as both the microvascular and macrovascular complications of diabetes. Infants receiving vitamin D supplements show as much as an 80 percent reduction in type I diabetes. (244)

In 2011 *Nature Reviews Immunology* published a review about the *Modulation of the immune system by UV radiation: more than just the effects of vitamin D?* Researchers show clearly that "vitamin D deficiencies are negatively related to insulin resistance and arterial stiffness. Diabetes combined with a vitamin D-deficient state doubles the relative risk of developing cardiovascular disease and mortality compared to diabetes with normal vitamin D levels." (245)

Gestational Diabetes and vitamin D

Diabetes during pregnancy affects about 5 percent of all pregnant women. (246) Gestational diabetes is increasing and may have deleterious effects on the fetus. Being overweight during pregnancy is an additional risk and may cause blood sugar disorders as well. Dr. Cuilin Zhang and colleagues at the NIH found women with low 25(OH)D levels were almost 3 times more likely to develop diabetes during pregnancy. (247)

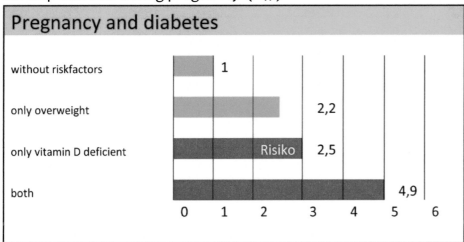

Foot problems caused by vitamin D deficiency

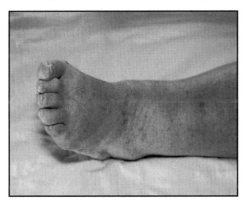

Many people with diabetes have peripheral arterial disease. The blood flow to finer capillaries in the feet is reduced causing nerve irritations and reduced sensation. This often leads to the typical painful foot problems, called diabetic foot and includes hard healing open wounds. In serious cases the foot has to be amputated.

The picture shows a strongly deformed foot. The clinic diagnosed it as diabetic foot and began treating the patient for diabetes. Despite treatment the symptoms increased. The patient then consulted Dr. von Helden, German physician. He was diagnosed with a severe vitamin D deficiency. After administering subsequent high level vitamin D over the next six months the complaints vanished. (248)

In April of 2012, Dr. Shalbha Tiwari and colleagues from the Banaras Hindu University in India wanted to know the prevalence and severity of vitamin D deficiency in patients with diabetic foot infection. The study concluded that "vitamin D deficiency was more prevalent and severe in patients with a diabetic foot infection. This study spurs the issue of recognizing severe vitamin D deficiency (< 25 nmol/l) as a possible risk factor for diabetic foot." (249)

Decreased cholesterol levels with vitamin D

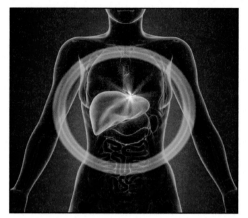

Nearly a third of American adults have high cholesterol, according to the Centers for Disease Control and Prevention. Cholesterol is vital. This delicate waxy substance is lifesaving. It is essential for cell membranes, hormones, vitamin D, and bile acids helping to digest fat. Cholesterol is a precursor to vitamin D. If this synthesis is obstructed, cholesterol will also inhibit the synthesis of vitamin D. (250)

Cholesterol also helps in the formation of memories and is vital for neurological function.

The metabolic pathways of vitamin D and cholesterol both run through the liver. The substances have the same origin: Both are made from 7-dehydrocholesterol.

The connection between vitamin D and cholesterol

The scientists of the Sunlight Research Forum researching on the impact of UV radiation on the human body have succeeded in establishing a link between vitamin D and cholesterol.

Researchers studied the habits of 177 Spanish participants. Their age ranges between 18 and 84 years. Once their vitamin D levels in blood tests were analyzed, a connection could be established between people working out doors or indoors. People working outdoors spent more time in the sun and had lower cholesterol levels and higher vitamin D levels. (251)

Research done in 2014 found that combining calcium and vitamin D supplements improved cholesterol levels in postmenopausal overweight or obese women. (251)

Clinical trial finds vitamin D supplementation increase the "good" cholesterol in children. (252)

Cancer and Vitamin D

All 700 billion cells in our bodies have certain jobs to do. Normal cells divide in an orderly way. They die when they are worn out or damaged and new cells take their place. Cancer is when the cells start to grow out of control. This causes problems in this part of the body and may lead to different types of cancer.

The connection between vitamin D and cancer

Vitamin D

- controls cell division, cell growth, cell death and cell cycle,
- supports functional cell to cell communication,
- enables the cells to recognize malignant cells and dispose of them, (253)

- acts as an immune system modulator,
- prevents excessive production of inflammatory cytokines and increases macrophage activity,
- stimulates the production of potent anti-microbial peptides in other white blood cells and in epithelial cells lining the respiratory tract,
- protects the organs from infection. (140)

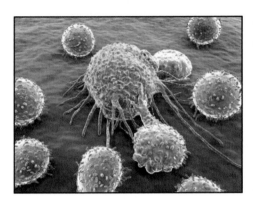

"We have determined the quantity of adequate amounts of vitamin D to prevent all types of invasive cancers, which had been unknown until the publication of this paper," said Cedric Garland in 2016, researcher and adjunct professor at the UC San Diego School of Medicine, Department of Family Medicine and Public Health. He concluded that optimal levels of vitamin D for cancer prevention, "are between 40 and 60 ng/ml. Most cancers occur in people with vitamin D blood levels between 10 and 40 ng/ml." (254)

According to the American Cancer Research Center National Cancer Institute, 80 percent of all cancer cases can be avoided. A study involving 1,179 healthy women from rural Nebraska showed that, "vitamin D and calcium supplementation reduces the risk of cancer by 77 percent." (255)

In 2011, a study carried out in France with 60,000 women after menopause, "showed a significantly lower risk of breast cancer in women who had particularly high vitamin D levels. This improved considerably when the women were actually exposed to sunlight." (256)

A landmark study done in 2016 found that, "women over 55 with blood concentrations of vitamin D higher than 40 ng/ml, had a 67 percent lower risk of cancer compared to women with levels lower than 20 ng/ml." (257)

Many cancers are thought to be more common with vitamin D deficiency. There is much convincing epidemiological and especially ecological evidence for this. (258)

Prostate cancer and vitamin D
Prostate cancer is the development of cancer in the prostate, a gland in the male reproductive system. Most prostate cancers grow slowly. The cancer cells may spread from the prostate to other parts of the body, particularly the bone-and lymph nodes.

The disease is responsible for about ten percent of deaths from cancer and thus represents the third leading cause of cancer death in men.

The connection between vitamin D and cancer of the prostate
An investigation of men undergoing surgery to remove a cancerous prostate show there is a link between low levels of vitamin D and the aggressiveness of this disease.

Lead investigator Adam Murphy, an assistant professor of urology, says: "Men with dark skin, low vitamin D intake or low sun exposure should be tested for vitamin D deficiency when they are diagnosed with an elevated PSA or prostate cancer. This deficiency should be corrected with supplements." (259)

The men with an aggressive prostate cancer had an average vitamin D level of 22.7 ng/ml. This is lower than the 30 ng/ml considered as normal.

Further findings suggest that, "prostate tumors in particular can become highly aggressive when the vitamin D level is rather low. A report done in 2014 in the journal *Clinical Cancer Research* showed that the lower the vitamin D level, the more aggressive the prostate cancer." (260)

"Vitamin D is important to several areas of health, cancer reduction being one of them," says prostate cancer expert Dr. Marc Garnick, Professor of Medicine at Harvard-affiliated Beth Israel Deaconess Medical Center and editor in chief of Harvard's Annual Report on Prostate Diseases. "In my practice, vitamin D, and if necessary, supplemental calcium in appropriate doses is generally a sound recommendation to consider." (261)

Risk of breast cancer is lower with vitamin D

Breast cancer is the most common invasive cancer in women worldwide. Researchers established

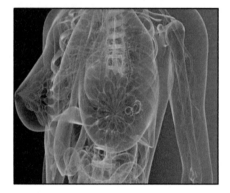

an overview and found that breast cancer, "accounts for 16 percent of all female cancers and 22.9 percent of invasive cancers in women. 18.2 percent of all cancer deaths worldwide, including both males and females, are from breast cancer." (262)

Breast cancer rates are much higher in developed nations compared to lower developing ones. The highest incidence of breast cancer was in Northern America and the lowest incidence in Asia and Africa.

The connection of vitamin D and breast cancer

There is growing evidence that solar UVB reduces the risk of breast and other cancers. (263) The global regions with higher cancer risks are similar to one with MS occurrences. People who live in sunnier regions of low- to mid-latitude countries have lower breast cancer and/or mortality rates than those living in the higher latitudes. For example, in the United States, the lowest breast cancer mortality rates are in Arizona, New Mexico, and Utah, while the highest rates are in the New England states. (264).

A 2005 study found that, "women with blood concentrations of vitamin D higher than 60 ng/ml had an 83 percent reduction in breast cancer compared with those lower than 20 ng/ml. Many holistic doctors and experts recommend that cancer patients aim for the 60-80 ng/ml range." (265)

In 2016 a study was published researching the *Effects of vitamin D and calcium supplementation on the side effects in patients of breast cancer treated with Letrozole.* It is no surprise that, "Aromatase inhibitors (AI) suppress estrogen levels in postmenopausal women with breast cancer by inhibiting the enzyme that activates estrogen production in fat tissue. Letrozole is a type of AI used in breast cancer hormone therapy treatment. Previous studies have shown that musculoskeletal symptoms worsened in patients taking Letrozole as a result of vitamin D deficiency and decreased estrogen production." The researchers concluded that in, "patients with breast cancer undergoing Letrozole treatment, vitamin D supplementation should be administered to those with insufficient levels. This would compensate for the declining levels." (266)

A study published at breastcancer.org suggests, "that women with low levels of vitamin D have a higher risk of breast cancer. Vitamin D may play a role in controlling normal breast cell growth. A vitamin D supplementation might even be able to stop breast cancer cells from developing." (267)

Risk of pancreatic cancer reduced with vitamin D

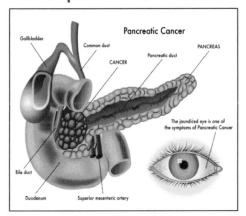

The pancreas is an abdominal gland organ. It is located behind the stomach and is surrounded by other organs, including the spleen, liver and small intestine. Several major blood vessels surround the pancreas. It produces enzymes, or digestive juices that are secreted into the small intestine to further break down food after it has left the stomach. The gland also produces the hormone insulin and secretes it into the blood stream in order to regulate the body's glucose or sugar level.

Pancreatic cancer is cancer of the pancreas. Approximately 44,000 people in the United States are diagnosed with pancreatic cancer every year. In Europe, more than 60,000 people are diagnosed with this disease each year. (268)

The connection between vitamin D and pancreatic cancer
Two Harvard studies found a correlation between vitamin D and pancreatic cancer:
- One 2009 study compared people, "taking 150 vs 600 international units (IU) (3.8 vs 15 mcg) vitamin D per day. There was a 40 percent lower cancer risk in people who took more vitamin D." (269)
- The other 2009 study found, "a 35 percent lower risk for those with higher vitamin D blood levels." (269)

A 2016 study conducted by Chen Yuan from the Dana-Farber Cancer Institute in Boston found, "that optimum serum 25(OH)D concentrations are associated with longer survival rates in pancreatic cancer patients." (270)

Colon cancer reduced with vitamin D

Colorectal cancer, also called colon cancer, rectal cancer or bowel cancer generally occurs in the large bowel. Cancer of the small bowel is rare. The World Health Organization says it is the second most common cancer worldwide, after lung cancer.

The connection between vitamin D and colorectal cancer

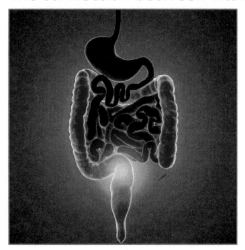

Over two decades ago, researchers first recognized the importance of vitamin D from sunlight in preventing colorectal cancer. They observed, "significantly higher mortality rates from colorectal cancer in the northern and northeastern United States, compared to the southwest, Hawaii, and Florida. In these sunnier climates individuals have a higher vitamin D level. People with higher levels of serum vitamin D had lower rates of colon cancer." (271)

The results of the meta-analysis revealed that, "by raising the serum level of vitamin D to 34 ng/ml, the rates of colorectal cancer could be reduced by half. Even higher levels of serum Vitamin D further reduced the colorectal cancer risk." As head researcher Edward Gorham, Ph.D. reported, "we project a two-thirds reduction of occurrence with serum levels of 46 ng/ml. This corresponds to a daily intake of 2,000 IU of vitamin D3. This could be best achieved through a combination of diet, supplements, and 10 to 15 minutes per day in the sun." (272)

Vitamin D may boost colon cancer survival, a study finds: "We found that patients who had vitamin D levels at the highest category had improved progression-free survival, compared with patients in the lowest category," said in 2015 lead author Dr. Kimmie Ng, an assistant professor of medicine at Harvard Medical School in Boston. (273)

A paper published in 2011 looked at 9 different studies involving vitamin D levels and the risk of developing colon or rectal cancer later in life. The researchers concluded, "People with the highest levels of vitamin D in their body had a 50 percent lower chance of developing rectal cancer, and a 23 percent lower chance of developing colon cancer than people with the lowest levels of vitamin D. There was a stronger link between vitamin D and rectal cancer than vitamin D and colon cancer." (274)

Colitis risks reduced with vitamin D

Ulcerative colitis is a relapsing form of inflammatory bowel disease that is characterized by chronic inflammation of the colon. Typical symptoms of colitis are frequent bloody-mucous diarrhea, often abdominal pain in the lower left abdomen, constant urging to stool, fever, general physical weakness and weight loss. Anemia and an abnormally fast heart rate have been witnessed in severe cases. (275)

Connection between vitamin D and colitis

Low vitamin D levels correlate to increased activity in ulcerative colitis. Research has also shown that, "a vitamin D deficiency is highly prevalent in both Crohn's disease and ulcerative colitis. Additionally, scientists have linked the effects of vitamin D supplementation with the disease severity and relapse in patients with inflammatory bowel disease." (276)

A 2016 study researched how *low vitamin D levels may increase the risk of ulcerative colitis relapse*. Researcher confirmed, "that higher vitamin D levels may reduce the risk of relapse in ulcerative colitis patients." (277)

Hair loss through chemotherapy may be prevented with Vitamin D

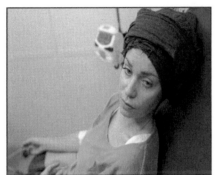

Vitamin D has effects in all areas where cell division plays an important role. It is of course equally important for the fastest regenerating cells, the cells of the skin and hair. Vitamin D has long been proven effective in cases of psoriasis and eczema. Vitamin D can obviously protect against hair loss resulting from chemotherapy. (278)

Vitamin D enhances stem cells growth and correct proliferation. Stem cells in the bulge of the hair follicle provide keratinocytes not only for hair follicle formation but also for the reepithelialization of the epidermis following chemotherapy. The function of these bulge stem cells is regulated by a vitamin D nuclear receptor.

All types of cancer are evidently related to insufficient vitamin D intake or production. (279) Inadequate vitamin D levels are therefore associated with ovarian cancer (280), polycystic ovary syndrome, (281) rheumatoid arthritis, (282) and lupus. (283)

A Medline search revealed nearly 300 papers on fighting prostate cancer with vitamin D and its derivatives, and nearly 400 in relation to vitamin D and breast cancer. (284)

Vitamin D may lead to a higher survival rate

One study published in July 2014 showed that "cancer patients with higher vitamin D levels had better chances for survival and remained in remission longer than patients with a vitamin D deficiency (below 75 nmol / l or below 30 ng / ml)." (285)

Creative Life and Vitamin D

We are born to live our life openly and completely,
Gaining new experiences,
Unfolding our potential.

Pregnancy and vitamin D

Vitamin D's role in pregnancy is an exciting field. It is biologically possible that vitamin D plays a role in pregnancy outcomes. Vitamin receptors are found in gestational tissues. Vitamin D receptors in uterine muscle could affect contractile strength. Woman Health published a 2012 research paper which speaks of the immunomodulatory effects of Vitamin D. This acts as a potential protection against infections for the host. (286)

- Vitamin D found in amniotic fluid may be due to a regulatory mechanism responding to the increased fetal demand for calcium in the final stages of pregnancy. (287)
- A recent randomized controlled trial has provided more evidence that vitamin D supplementation reduces the risk of maternal comorbidities and improves the health of infants. (288)
- Research suggests vitamin D supplementation reduces depression during pregnancy. (289)
- A study ascertains that vitamin D supplementation during pregnancy helps reduce childhood allergies. (290)
- Lower levels of vitamin D have been associated with increased rates of Caesarean section delivery. (291)
- Higher levels of vitamin D regulate the glucose metabolism efficiently of mother and child. (292)
- Sufficient vitamin D levels during pregnancy reduce the risk of allergies and asthma in the offspring. (293)
- Iranian researchers show that pregnant women with multiple sclerosis benefit from taking 50,000 IU/week of vitamin D3. (294)
- Vitamin D status during late pregnancy may relate to the infant language development. (295)
- A study finds vitamin D levels during pregnancy may relate to the dental health in children. (296)
- The risk of gestational diabetes can be reduced with vitamin D. (297)
- A further study shows 4,000 IU a Day of Vitamin D may reduce preterm birth and other risks. (298)
- Pregnant mothers with high levels of vitamin D have a higher chance of a child with higher IQ. (299)
- Babies score higher on development tests if their moms get enough vitamin D during pregnancy, according to a Spanish study. (300)

The connection between vitamin D and pregnancy

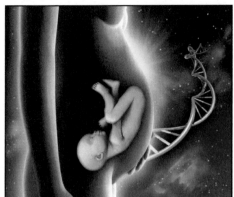

In the last years, an increasing amount of research concludes that some of the damage done by Vitamin D deficiency is done *in utero*, while the fetus is developing. This research points out that, "a vitamin D deficiency during pregnancy endangers the mother's life and health, and is the cause of future perils for the child, especially for the child's brain and immune system." (301)

Dr. Lisa Bodnar, a prolific Vitamin D researcher, and her colleagues at the University of Pittsburg studied 400 pregnant Pennsylvania women: "63 percent had levels below 30 ng/ml. 44 percent of the black women in the study had levels below 15 ng/ml. Prenatal vitamins had little effect on the deficiency." (301)

Dr. Dijkstra and his colleagues studied 70 pregnant women in the Netherlands, "none had levels above 40 ng/ml and 50 percent had levels below 10 ng/ml. Again, prenatal vitamins appeared to have little effect on 25(OH)D levels, as prenatal vitamins contain only 400 IU of Vitamin D. More than 95 percent of pregnant women had 25(OH)D levels below 50 ng/ml, the level that may indicate chronic substrate starvation." (302)

Effects on mother and child

Caesarean section
The rate of Caesarean section in American women has increased from 5 percent in 1970 to 30 percent today. Dr. Anne Merewood and her colleagues at Boston University School of Medicine found women with, "levels below 15 ng/ml were four times more likely to have a Caesarean section than women with higher levels." (303)

Preeclampsia
Preeclampsia is a common obstetrical condition in which hypertension is combined with excess protein in the urine. This could be life-threatening for the mother and the baby. Dr. Lisa Bodnar and her colleagues found women, "with 25(OH)D levels less than 15 ng/mL had a five-fold increase in the risk of preeclampsia." (304)

Bacterial Vaginitis
Dr. Lisa Bodnar and her colleagues found pregnant women, "with the lowest 25(OH)D level were almost twice as likely to get a bacterial vaginal infection during their pregnancy." (302)

Birth weight
The total intake of Vitamin D was associated with increased infant birth weight. "Pregnant mothers below the current adequate intake (<5 µg/day or 200 IU) had infants with significantly lower birth weights. Additional intake of Vitamin D may be of importance since a higher intake is associated with increased birth weight in a population at risk of adverse pregnancy outcomes." (305)

Eye sight improved with vitamin D

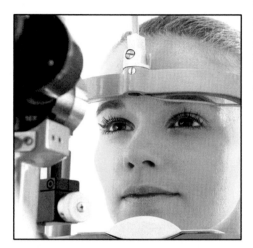

Vitamin D protects eyes from premature ageing, including inflammation. (306) Boosting vitamin D intake could help prevent deteriorating eyesight and blindness in older people. Scientists said "tests revealed taking vitamin D for six weeks could improve vision in middle-aged subjects." (307)

Lead scientist Professor Glen Jeffery, from the University College London stated in 2012, "There is growing evidence that many of us in the western world are deficient in vitamin D and this could be having significant health implications. Age-related inflammation and damage to the eye's retina can lead to macular degeneration, the biggest cause of blindness in people over the age of 50 in the developed world." (308)

A 2012 study funded by the *Biotechnology and Biological Sciences Research Council* (BBSRC) discovered a link between vitamin D and eyesight. (309)

Several studies credited the improvement in eyesight to:
- Reduction in macrophages. Macrophages normally fight off infection in our bodies. Misguided macrophages can actually cause harm to eyes. Vitamin D supplementation reduced the number of damaging macrophages and activated healthy macrophages. (309)
- Reduction in amyloid beta. Amyloid beta is a toxin that collects in our bodies as we age. As the amount of it increases, our risk for age-related macular degenerations also increases. Vitamin D supplementation caused a reduction in the deposits of amyloid beta. (309)
- Studies in 2012 linked vitamin D to protection against age-related macular degeneration. Hence, vitamin D (3) enrichment is likely to represent a beneficial route for those at risk. (310)

Athletes improved with vitamin D

Vitamin D is important to athletes, affecting bone mass, immunity, endurance and physical performance. This study evaluated the prevalence of vitamin D insufficiency in young athletes and dancers. A high prevalence of vitamin D insufficiency was identified with young athletes and dancers from various disciplines in sunny countries. (311)

Alexander Martens, a German graduate of sport sciences wrote in his thesis, "Vitamin D increases the protein synthesis. This in turn leads to a faster and more effective increase in intra- and intermuscular coordination. In the maximum oxygen intake, that is the maximum amount of oxygen per minute that average athlete can consume during a sporting exercise, it could be demonstrated that vitamin D levels above 30 ng/ml lead to a significant increase in maximal oxygen

intake, thus improved performance and lowered the risk of injury." Martens believes an athletic body requires a daily intake of 6,000 IU.

A 2016 study published by the Orthopedic Journal of Sports Medicine suggests that "nearly 80 percent of professional basketball players have inadequate vitamin D levels." (312)

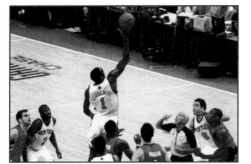

Vitamin D in athletic performance is linked to an improved vertical jump height, exercise capacity and sprint times. This is further revealed by a randomized controlled trial determining that vitamin D supplementation increases type 2 muscle fiber size. Type 2 muscle fibers are responsible for fast, powerful movements.

Dr. John Cannell reveals in his book Faster *Quicker Stronger* that vitamin D supplementation has been a long-held secret used mainly by eastern European athletic trainers. Vitamin D, the sunshine vitamin, improves muscle tone, muscle strength, balance, reaction time and physical endurance, as well as immunity and general health. It has applications ranging from improved performance of standing armies in the field, to Olympic and every-day athletes, and even seniors who need to avert falls and age-related loss of muscle mass and muscle tone. (313)

Lifespan and protein homeostasis enhanced with vitamin D

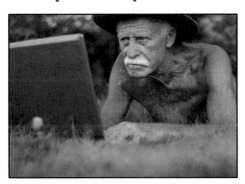

A new animal study published in 2016 in the journal *Cell Reports* (314) shows that vitamin D, "engages longevity genes to increase their lifespan and prevent the accumulation of toxic proteins linked to age-related chronic diseases." (315)

Research in 2016 at the Buck Institute shows that vitamin D, "works through genes known to influence longevity and impacts processes associated with many human age-related diseases." The study, published in *Cell Reports*, explains why vitamin D deficiency has been linked to breast, colon and prostate cancer, as well as obesity, heart disease, and depression. (316)

Vitamin D acting in longevity genes, "extended median lifespan by 33 percent and slowed the aging-related misfolding of hundreds of proteins in the worm," said Gordon Lithgow, PhD, senior author and Buck Institute professor. "Our findings provide a real connection between aging and disease and give clinicians and other researchers an opportunity to look at vitamin D in a much larger context." (314)

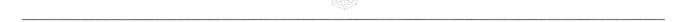

Older people live better with vitamin D

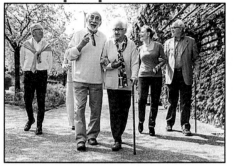

Aging slows down the metabolic processes, and it also leads to a reduced ability to produce Vitamin D in the skin. A 70-year-old who is exposed to the same dose of sunlight as a 20-year-old produces only about 25 percent of vitamin D3, which a 20-year-old can produce. (317)

Inadequate amounts of vitamin D in older people reduce wellbeing and aggravate the ageing process. In particular insufficiency, "reduces mobility and adds to the severity of osteoporosis and the risks of falls and fragility fractures with all of their severe consequences." (318)

A 2010 study showed that the vitamin D status is especially low in elderly women. Alarmingly low levels of vitamin D have been found especially in nursing home residents. (319)

Adequate vitamin D levels may enhance longevity, reduce the risk of cardiovascular disease and reduce the risks of type 2 diabetes and certain common cancers, notably colorectal cancer. (318)

Pineal gland decalcified through vitamin D

A pine cone shaped gland located in the center of the brain, the pineal gland is about the size of a small pea. It has one of the body's most abundant blood supplies. Only the kidneys carry more

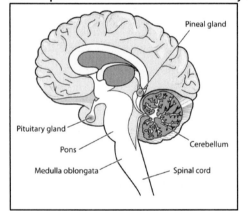

oxygenating blood. The pineal gland produces melatonin, a serotonin derived hormone which modulates sleep patterns in both circadian and seasonal cycles.

Studies done in 1988 showed that vitamin D and the pineal hormones are messengers with comprehensive actions on endocrine, autonomic, sensory, skeletal, and motor functions. "In a complementary fashion, both hormone systems appear to correlate biological activities with the daily and seasonal changes of our solar environment." (320)

Pineal calcification occurs in an estimated 40 percent of Americans by the age of 17. Two-thirds of the entire adult population has it. Research shows that Alzheimer's patients have more pineal calcification than people with other forms of dementia. They are usually also deficient in melatonin and vitamin D. (321)

Vitamin D is a fat-soluble nutrient that functions much like a hormone in the body to regulate calcium metabolism. It has been known to decalcify the pineal gland. (322)

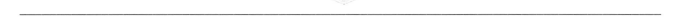

Longevity and vitamin D

Let's get back to the foundations, to the first omnipotent stem cell of our genetic body. The structure that contains the cell's genetic material is a chromosome. That genetic material determines how an organism develops. It is a molecule of deoxyribonucleic acid (DNA). This DNA is tightly packed in long chains of associated proteins.

In 1975–1977, Elizabeth Blackburn, working as a postdoctoral fellow at Yale University with Joseph Gall, discovered the unusual nature of telomeres, with their simple repeated DNA sequences composing chromosome ends. In 1930 Muller named these

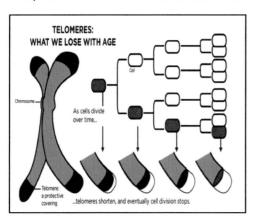

sealing ends telomeres. Its name is derived from the Greek nouns telos (τέλος) "end" and meros (μέρος, root: μερ-) "part." "Telomeres contain an array of highly repeated DNA sequences and specific binding proteins." (323) The most prominent function of the telomeres is to protect chromosome ends against degradation and fusion with neighboring chromosomes. Telomeres are of great importance for rejuvenation.

Source: www.glymedplus.com

"Telomeres are responsible for maintaining genomic integrity" as researchers confirm. (324)

Each time a cell divides, its telomeres become shorter. After years of splicing and dicing, telomeres are too short for any more divisions. At this point, the cells are unable to divide any further and become inactive, die or continue dividing anyway. This is an abnormal process which is potentially dangerous.

in 2014 study, scientists concluded that an, "accelerated telomere loss has been associated with many chronic diseases of aging. Short telomeres, for example, are associated with a wide variety of conditions including osteoporosis, heart failure, cancer, hypertension and dementia." (324)

Telomerase is an enzyme that lengthens telomeres and keeps them from wearing out too fast or too early. With constant cell division, telomerase levels are depleted. (325)

The connection between vitamin D and telomerase

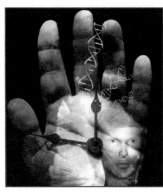

A survey done 2016 studied the association of telomere length and serum 25-hydroxyvitamin D levels in US adults. The *National Health and Nutrition Examination Survey* supports, "a possible positive association between 25(OH)D levels and telomere length." (326)

In 2007, 2,160 women in the United Kingdom participated in a study to examine the effect between higher serum vitamin D concentrations and longer leukocyte telomere length. A longer leucocyte telomere length comes with increased serum vitamin D concentrations. It is known that vitamin D generation decelerates with age, as well as leucocyte telomere length. These markers are regarded as aging signals. The researchers have shown, "that the positive association between leucocyte telomere length and vitamin D concentrations is independent of age and many other variables." (327)

In fact, a study done on mice showed the premature aging effect when lacking telomerase. But when the enzyme was replaced, the mice bounced back to health. (328) By regenerating telomerase in human cells, normal human aging could be slowed. "This has implications for thinking about telomerase as a serious anti-aging intervention," said Ronald DePinho, a cancer geneticist who led the study. (329)

Scientists at the Georgia Health Sciences University, led by Dr. Zhu reported on the effect of vitamin D on telomerase activity in obese African Americans. The authors found that vitamin D increased telomerase activity by 19 percent. (330)

DNA the Blueprint of Life and Vitamin D

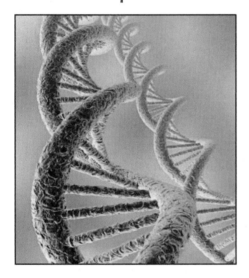

DNA is important in terms of our genetic code. It transfers genetic messages to all of the cells in our body. This is the code our body uses for our entire life. (331) DNA is frequently called the "blueprint" of an organism.

DNA repair is a combination of step by step processes. The cell identifies the damage to the DNA, initiates a comprehensive repair mechanism. Damages can occur both through normal metabolic activities and environmental factors such as radiation. These environmental factors are multifaceted and correlated to the individual's present intoxication status. "This results in up to a million individual DNA lesions per cell per day." (332)

The connection between vitamin D and DNA
Studies using genes expression profiling revealed that the, "DNA repairing genes are among a multitude of genes whose transcription is induced by activated vitamin D. The role of vitamin D can be divided into a primary function that prevents damage in DNA and a secondary function that regulates the growth rate of cells." (333)

- There is ample evidence that activated vitamin D provides protection against oxidative DNA damage.
- Activated vitamin D directly upregulates a key antioxidant, thioredoxin reductase. (334)
- Antioxidant protein superoxide dismutase is induced by activated vitamin D. (334)
- The authors found that activated vitamin D lessened the DNA damage in colon cells. (335)
- There is evidence that vitamin D regulates genes for proteins that protect the genome. (336)

- It is possible that vitamin D directly controls the expression of a variety of genes whose protein products are involved in DNA damage repair and programmed cell death, thereby offering protection against carcinogenesis. (336)

DNA repair is essential for the survival and longevity of our species. Such repair or change also helps ensure that one lives up to his/her full potential in this world.

Stem Cells and Vitamin D

History
Since the 19th century, scientists from all over the world have studied stem cells, from every living being starting from plants to mice, and further to individual people in search for a cure for diseases. (337)

1868 – The term "stem cell" appears in scientific literature. The German biologist Ernst Haeckel uses stem cell to describe the fertilized egg that carries all the DNA specifications to become an organism. The single-celled organism acting as the ancestor cell to all living things in history was called a stem cell. (338)

1909 – Russian academic Alexander Maximow lectures at the Berlin Hematological Society on a theory that all blood cells come from the same ancestor cell. This introduces the idea of multi-potent blood stem cells, or cells with the ability to differentiate into several types of cells. (339)

1957 – Donnall Thomas, a physician-scientist working in Seattle, attempts the first human bone marrow transplantation. He is awarded the Nobel Prize for his research work in 1990. (340)

1968 – Robert A. Good of the University of Minnesota performs the first successful bone marrow transplant on a child patient suffering from an immune deficiency. The boy received bone marrow from his sister, and he grew into healthy adulthood. (337)

1981 – Two scientists, Martin Evans of the University of Cambridge and Gail Martin of the University of California, San Francisco, conduct separate studies. They derived totipotent stem cells from the embryos of mice. These early cells are the first embryonic stem cells ever to be isolated. (338)

1988 – The first cord blood transplant was performed in a patient with Fanconi anemia. The umbilical cord blood was collected and cryopreserved at birth. The transplant was successful and the patient is currently alive and free of disease more than 15 years after transplant, with full hematologic and immunologic donor reconstitution. (341)

1992 – Pablo Rubinstein establishes the world's first public cord blood bank in New York. An inventory of cord blood units is built up for patients in need of a stem cell match from a public registry. (338)

2008 – The Stem Cell Program at Boston Children's Hospital announces the creation of 10 disease-specific lines of stem cells. (337)

2009 –The FDA (US Food and Drug Administration) approves cord blood-derived hematopoietic progenitor cells (blood forming stem cells) for certain applications. The FDA has not approved any other stem cell-based products for usage. (342)

2007 – Researchers led by Dr. Anthony Atala claimed that a new type of stem cell had been isolated in amniotic fluid. (343)

2011 – Cord blood use increases. The amount of cord blood transplants has quadrupled. More than 30,000 transplants have been performed worldwide.

2016 – There are over 1,358 clinical trials investigating the application of cord blood in medicine. (344) In addition, there are over 5,000 clinical trials investigating the role of stem cells. Discoveries from these trials influenced cord blood research and the application of cord blood. (345)

A magical stem cell gives birth to a human body

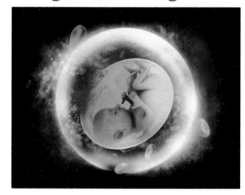

The twenty-three chromosomes from the father's side interlock with twenty-three chromosomes from the mother's side when a single celled sperm and egg unite. Instantly a uniquely powerful stem cell is created. Science calls this a zygote cell. This cell is totipotent. It is the first genetic blueprint for every subsequent cell in the body. Within several days, these totipotent cells divide and create even more totipotent cells. After approximately four days the cells begin to specialize into pluripotent cells, which can go on to specialize further.

Virtually all human cells, such as nerve or heart cells, the cartilage and ligaments, the skin and bones, all precious organs and fluids, and 100 billion interconnected neurons in the brain are created out of this first magic cell.

Potent stem cells

Stem cells are often called "master cells" because they are unspecialized cells that develop into specialized cells in the body's tissues and organs.

Stem cells are cells that have the potential to mature into myriad different cell types in the body. Stem cells can be totipotent, pluripotent, or multipotent. This determines their operational activity. They can theoretically divide without limits to replenish other cells for as long as the person or animal is still alive. For example, the stem cells in the hippocampus region of the brain burst out into neuronal cells; stem cells in the bone marrow create special blood cells or immune cells.

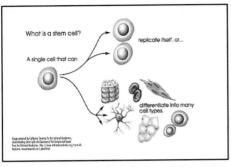

Source: www.nationalmssociety.org

The DNA information of the stem cell is encoded, yet only one part is necessary for an active blood cell. According to the National Institute for Health, stem cells serve as a sort of repair system for the body. (347) Stem cells play a pivotal role in the modern treatment of diseases including macular degeneration, spinal cord injury, stroke, burns, heart disease, diabetes, osteoarthritis, rheumatoid arthritis, many forms of cancer and more. (348)

Stem cells are nature's pharmacy and they are usually found in bone marrow, brain, adipose fat, blood vessels, skeletal muscle, skin, heart, liver and more. They are responsible for healthy cellular and tissue growth. When a stem cell divides (mitosis), each daughter cell comes with the potential to stay a stem cell or to become another cell with a more specialized function. (349)

Stem cells differ from other kinds of cells in the body. All stem cells – regardless of their source – have three general properties:
- they are capable of dividing and renewing themselves even after long periods of inactivity,
- they are unspecialized,
- they can transform into specialized cell types,
- they can be induced to become tissue- or organ-specific cells with special functions.

Stem cells may be totipotent, pluripotent or multipotent.
- A fertilized egg is a totipotent stem cell and as such can develop into any specialized cell found in the organism. It is during the early cell divisions in embryonic development that more totipotent cells are produced. Within several days, these totipotent cells divide and create replicas, therefore producing more totipotent cells. It is after approximately four days that the cells begin to specialize into pluripotent cells, which can go on to specialize further but can't ever produce an entire organism as totipotent cells can. (350)
- Pluripotent stem cells can transmute into any type of cell in the body except those needed to support and develop a fetus in the womb. Embryonic cells and the cord blood stem cells are pluripotent. (351)
- Multipotent cells can develop into more than one cell type, but are more limited than pluripotent cells; adult stem cells (somatic stem cells) are considered multipotent. (352)

Adult or somatic stem cells
An adult or somatic stem cell is an undifferentiated cell, found in various cells in a tissue or organ. The adult stem cell can renew itself and can differentiate to produce any of the major specialized cell types of the tissues or organs. Adult stem cells have their primary function to repair and regenerate the system in which they are found. They are multipotent. They have been identified in many organs and tissues, including brain, bone marrow, peripheral blood, blood vessels, skeletal muscle, skin, teeth, heart, gut, liver, ovarian epithelium, and testicles. (353)

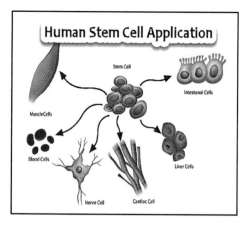

Adult or somatic stem cells carry the memory of this special person with their entire health history. Georg Siegel and a team of researchers stated in 2013, "Phenotype, donor age and gender affect the function of human bone marrow-derived mesenchymal stromal cells." (354)

Cord blood stem cells

Cord blood comes from a newborn's umbilical cord and is collected immediately after birth. The baby's umbilical cord comprised of tissue and contains blood. Both cord blood and cord tissues are rich sources of powerful pluripotent stem cells. (355) Postnatal stem cells recovered from the umbilical cord, including the umbilical cord blood cells, amnion/placenta, umbilical cord vein, or umbilical cord matrix cells, are a readily available. (356)

Embryonic and fetal stem cells

Embryonic stem cells are gained by extracting cells from the early embryo. Once two cells unite into a zygote stem cell, the embryo begins up to 8 or 9 weeks its development. From this point on it is called a fetus. Embryonic stem cells are taken from embryos, whereby the embryo loses its life. Embryonic stem cells can be cultured in laboratory situations too. Both embryonic and fetal stem cells have been subject to ethical and scientific issues.

The connection between vitamin D and stem cells

A multitude of research and applications document the vital connection between vitamin D and stem cell research and treatment.

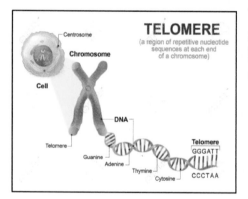

The life cycle of every cell is carefully controlled. Cells divide according to their function. The average body cell will divide between 50 and 70 times. As a cell divides, the telomeres on the end of the chromosome shorten.

Stem cells express an enzyme called telomerase that acts to lengthen the telomeres. This allows stem cells to divide many more times than most body cells. Vitamin D enhances this process.

Researchers find "telomere shortening occurs in most human somatic cells. This triggers DNA damage responses that mediate cell cycle arrest or apoptosis. Hematopoietic stem cells can escape this trigger by employing a telomerase-dependent telomere lengthening mechanism in replication." (357)

2012 – A study published to research *1,25-Dihydroxyvitamin D3 suppresses Telomerase Expression and Human Cancer Growth through MicroRNA* confirmed that even embryonic stem cells possess vitamin

D receptor sites. "This may have profound implications in aging and lifespan regulation. Vitamin D advances the current understanding about species-specific telomerase regulation. " (358)

2013 – A study was published to research the Role *of Vitamin D in Hematologic Disease and Stem Cell Transplantation*. Researchers concluded, "Ultimately, the ubiquity of the vitamin D receptor and the myriad physiologic effects that have been found suggest multiple mechanisms of potential benefit from the use of Vitamin D in the treatment of hematologic disease. In the hematopoietic system there is evidence that the vitamin D pathway affects both differentiation of cells and their ultimate activation. Similarly, immune-modulatory effects of vitamin D almost certainly affect the complicated immune environment in patients who have had allogeneic stem cell transplants." (359)

2014 – A study published researching *Vitamin D Levels Affect Outcome in Pediatric Hematopoietic Stem Cell Transplantation* comes to conclusion that, "in this study group the neutrophil granulocytes rose significantly faster in the vitamin D sufficient group. Vitamin D may have an important impact on the outcome of pediatric Hematopoietic stem cell transplantation, particularly in patients with malignant disease." (360)

2015 – A study published researching the *Role of vitamin D in regulating the neural stem cells of mouse model with multiple sclerosis* concludes that the, "lesion associated apoptotic signals are reduced when administrated with vitamin D. The present data helps to design a new therapeutic intervention to cure MS." (361)

2016 – A public release on how *Vitamin D increases the number of blood stem cells during embryonic development* states, "What was surprising was that Vitamin D is having an impact so early. We really only thought about Vitamin D in terms of bone development and maintenance, but we clearly show that, human blood stem cells can respond directly to this nutrient." (362)

2016 – *Stem Cells International* published a research article *Vitamin D Effects on Osteoblastic Differentiation of Mesenchymal Stem Cells from Dental Tissues*. Researchers conclude, "Our finding that vitamin D stimulates osteoblastic differentiation of Dental Bud Stem Cells with the subsequent increase of bone mineral matrix deposition suggests a possible use of vitamin D as food aid in reconstructive therapies of bone with adult stem cell treatments." (363)

Fountain of youth and vitamin D

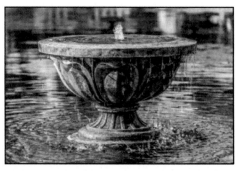

According to myth, the Spanish explorer Ponce de Leon was seeking the legendary Fountain of Youth when he landed on the coast of Florida in 1513. It has long been said that he who drinks from the fountain will be forever young.

In 2010 Dr. Denise Houston and J. Paul her team from the Sticht Center on Aging at Wake Forest University studied the relationship between vitamin D status and physical function in a group of relatively healthy seniors living in Memphis, TN and Pittsburgh, PA.

2,788 seniors with average age of 75 years were monitored for 4 years. The blood was analyzed and the vitamin D level charted. In the beginning of the study a better physical condition was seen in participants with the highest levels of 25-hydroxyvitamin D. After the 4-year interval and a final blood test, a significant increase in physical and mental activities had been documented. Participants with higher vitamin D levels were more active than participants with moderate levels. (364)

Answering the question whether vitamin D will be a Fountain of Youth, Jonny Bowden, MD answers, "probably not. But paying attention to how much vitamin D we get is important at every age and will help enhance the quality component of life as we enter our senior years. I believe this study just adds to the voluminous research indicating a need for much greater vitamin D intake than is now recommended. We've seen vitamin D associated with bone strength, improved mood, physical performance, even reduced rates of certain cancers. I think vitamin D is one of a very few supplements that virtually everyone could benefit from." (365)

Vitamins are substances needed by everybody to stay healthy. The only vitamin that our body can create on its own is vitamin D. Indeed, it is essential.

Vitamin D is the mediating essence for any type of cellular communication, regeneration, repair, modulation, nourishing, reforming, stabilizing and rejuvenation.

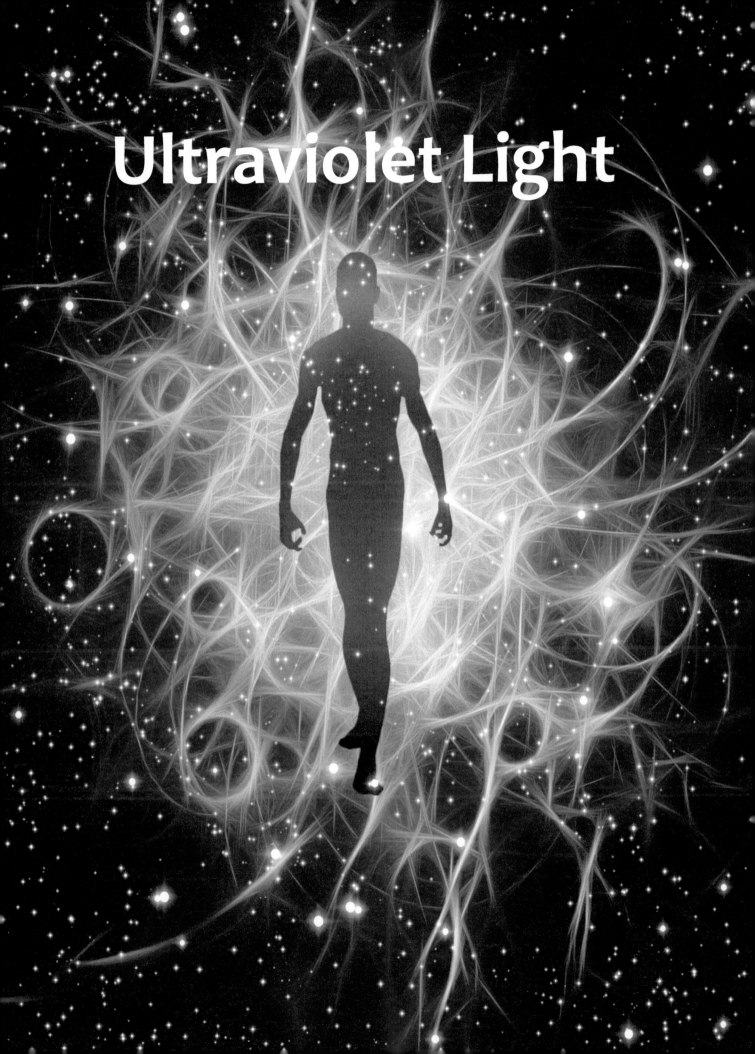

Chapter Four

Ultraviolet Light

The discovery of ultraviolet light

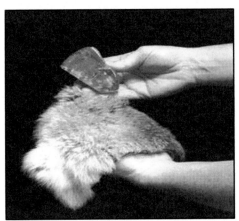

Source: www.newtonsapple.org.uk

At about 600 BC, the ancient Greek philosopher Thales of Miletus the discovered that rubbing fur on amber (fossilized tree resin) caused an attraction between the two. What he actually discovered was static electricity.

In 1600, English physician William Gilbert coined the word: "electric" (from the Greek word for amber). A few years later another English scientist, Thomas Browne used the word "electricity" to describe his investigations based on Gilbert's work. At this time, it was believed that electricity was only caused by friction.

In 1752, Ben Franklin conducted his experiment with a kite, a key, and a storm. The experiment's purpose was to uncover the unknown facts about the nature of lightning and electricity.

In 1800, Italian physicist Alessandro Volta invented the first electric battery – which people then called the "voltaic pile." Applying his invention, scientists were able to produce steady flows of electric current for the first time. This opened the door to new discoveries and technologies.

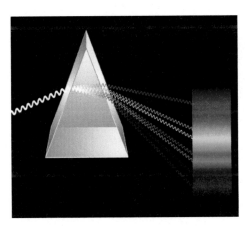

In 1800, a German astronomer, Fredrich William Herschel, was experimenting with sending sunlight through a glass prism. He observed that temperatures increased the more the rays neared the red end of the spectrum. As a scientist he measured beyond the red end of the spectrum, naming it "ultra-red."

A year later, Johann Wilhelm Ritter, Polish-born physicist, related to Herschel's ultra-red discovery, and proceeded with his own experiments at the University of Jena and detected "ultraviolet light" beyond the violet end of the spectrum (366)

Violet is the color of the highest frequency of visible light. Consequently, ultraviolet has a higher frequency than violet light.

In 1877 two English scientists, W. B. Hugo Downes and Thomas Porter Blunt, discovered that sunlight kills bacteria. An easy experiment led them to this discovery. They placed a vessel filled with sugar water so that one side was exposed to sunlight while the other side was constantly in the shade. The part in the sun remained clear while the other side grew obscure with bacteria. (367)

It wasn't until 1892 that Marshall Ward demonstrated that it was primarily the ultraviolet part of the spectrum that had the bacteria-killing properties.

This new discovery unleashed great potentials for new technologies. It did not take long for the first applications to appear on the market.

Ultraviolet light and its applications

UV light and clean drinking water
Ultraviolet disinfection of water has a long and well-proven history. UV light has long been accepted as an effective germicidal treatment, and has been installed in many major public drinking water and wastewater treatment plants worldwide.

In September 2006 St Petersburg, Russia opened the world's largest UV drinking water disinfection plant with a capacity of 2.5 million cubic meters per day. (368) This unique and rapid method of water disinfection uses neither heat nor chemicals. UV sterilizers utilize germicidal ultraviolet lamps that produce short wave radiation lethal to bacteria, viruses, and other microorganisms present in water.

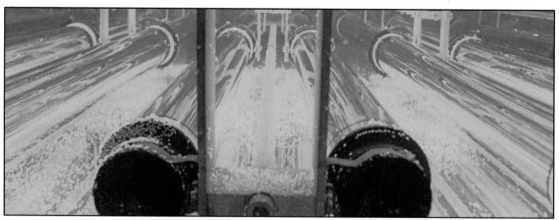
Source: www.waterworlds.com

UV light sanitizes air conditioners
Air-conditioning systems work very well to cool rooms. but quite often they fail to remove pollutants from the air. Air flows through a filtering system and is redistributed back into the room with a risk of recirculating various indoor allergens, dust, mold, or bacteria back into the room. The warmth and moisture found in the heating, ventilation, and air conditioning (HVAC) systems of households, hospitals, and office buildings make the perfect breeding ground for airborne molds, microorganisms, and bacteria. Unlike filters which collect pollutants as they pass through the

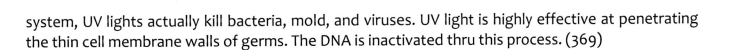

system, UV lights actually kill bacteria, mold, and viruses. UV light is highly effective at penetrating the thin cell membrane walls of germs. The DNA is inactivated thru this process. (369)

UV light in washing machines
A new invention was patented 2009 under patent application No. US 8303718 B2 for a "Sterilizable washing machine using ultraviolet radiation." (370) The washing system utilizes UVC light to clean nanocoated fabric.

UV light in tumble dryers
A tumble dryer has been designed to incorporate ultraviolet light sources. A series of ultraviolet emitters are located around the perimeter of the drying drum inside of the dryer. As the clothes dryer operates, these lamps are energized and their light passes into the drying drum. A patent was granted in 1997. (371) Such a dryer could be particularly useful in hospitals, in centers where biological studies are performed, or for individuals susceptible to infectious diseases.

UV light in dishwashers
Dirty dishes may carry a host of germs and bacteria. Designers incorporated a distinctive UV lamp to prevent bacterial growth and eradicate 99 percent of the bacteria remaining after a wash cycle. The UV lamp emits an ultraviolet light that damages bacteria DNA and halts their reproduction. In 2014 *Expert Reviews* presented one of these machines. (372)

UV light powered comb to treat psoriasis
An elegant phototherapy unit uses UVB light to treat psoriasis. It is specially equipped with a comb attachment with round bristles to remove scalp psoriasis more gently. The ultraviolet light goes directly through hair into the upper part of the scalp. A 2015 study proves this technology "lastly, NB-UVB appears to be a safe and effective treatment to be used alongside with biologic agents for recalcitrant psoriasis."

UV light brooms disinfects hospital floors

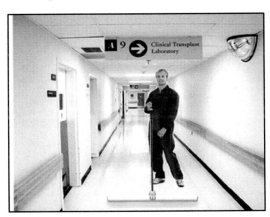

Source: www.mrsa-uv.com

MRSA (methicillin-resistant staphylococcus aureus), the "super-bug," is a harmful bacterium. It is resistant to numerous antibiotics including methicillin, amoxicillin, penicillin, and oxacillin. MRSA infections are a major cause of illness and death that also imposes serious economic costs on patients and hospitals.

MRSA can easily enter the body through feet or toes. UV lights are effectively used to sanitize hospital floors. "UV light will effectively pick up where chemicals leave off,"

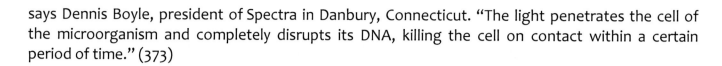

says Dennis Boyle, president of Spectra in Danbury, Connecticut. "The light penetrates the cell of the microorganism and completely disrupts its DNA, killing the cell on contact within a certain period of time." (373)

UV light emitting machine disinfects hospital rooms in minutes

Cooley Dickinson Hospital in Northampton, Massachusetts treats 40,000 emergency room patients a year. Antibiotic-resistant bacteria infect 100,000 patients annually and are notoriously hard to fight. One study by Dr. Roy Chemaly, head of infection control at Houston's MD Anderson Cancer Center, found "that even after swabbing with bleach, alcohol, and other biocides, 8 percent of high-touch surfaces like tray tables, door handles, and remote controls in hospitals still tested positively for superbugs." *Forbes Magazine* published the study in 2011. (374)

A device bathes hospital rooms with intense, millisecond pulses of ultraviolet light from a high-wattage strobe light. The UV penetrates bacteria and either scrambles their DNA or kills them outright. (375)

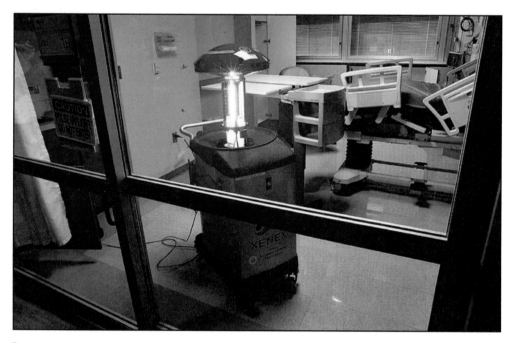

Source: ww.post-gazette.com

Ultraviolet light – a healing essence

Photoluminescence therapy cures illnesses

UV photoluminescence sounds high-tech, but it's actually simple. "Photo" means light and "luminescence" is emission of light. It is also called biophotonic therapy or UVBI (ultraviolet blood irradiation).

According to Dr. Ron Kennedy of Santa Rosa California, the advent of vaccines and antibiotics shunted photoluminescence therapy so far into the shadows of disuse that it was nearly forgotten.

But now he says with the, "dangers and lack of efficacy of vaccination alarmingly considered, the development of dangerous antibiotic resistant species of bacteria, and with the difficulty eradicating many viruses (including those involved in AIDS), photoluminescence has been reassessed as a viable alternative therapy." (376)

In 1892 Marshall Ward applied ultraviolet light to kill bacteria.

In 1903 Niels Finsen was awarded the Nobel Prize for his work on UV rays and various skin conditions. The success rates were 98 percent in thousands of cases, mostly for the treatment of lupus vulgaris. (377)

In June 1934 the first article on the benefit of phototherapy was published by Hancock and Knott. By June 1942, 6,520 patients had been treated with UV therapy. The treatment was successful for almost every case. No harmful side effects were reported. (378)

The dissertation by Virgil Hancock, M.D. and Emmet K. Knott listed the following experiences with photoluminescence therapy:

- Inactivation of toxins
- Destruction and inhibition of bacterial growth
- Oxygen increase combining efficacy of the blood and oxygen transportation to the organs
- stimulation of cellular and humoral (relating to bodily fluids) immunity (humoral immunity was a catchall phrase in a time before the complexities of the human immune system were understood)
- Vivication of steroid hormones
- Vasodilatation
- Activation of white blood cells
- Decreased platelet aggregation
- Stimulation of fibrinolysis (the breakdown of blood clots)
- Decreased viscosity of blood
- Stimulation of corticosteroid production
- Improved microcirculation (379)

In the 1940s, countless articles appeared in American literature specifying this unique treatment for infection. "This UV treatment had a cure rate of 98 to 100 percent in early and moderately advanced infections, and approximately 50 percent in terminally ill patients." Healing was not limited to just bacterial infections, but also wounds, asthma, arthritis, and viral infections such as acute polio. There were reports of good results in killing airborne pathogens. German literature revealed "profound improvements in a number of biochemical and hematologic markers." No toxic side effects, burns, or injury were ever documented. It was a treatment without administering costly pharmaceutical substances. (380)

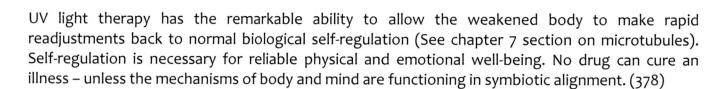

UV light therapy has the remarkable ability to allow the weakened body to make rapid readjustments back to normal biological self-regulation (See chapter 7 section on microtubules). Self-regulation is necessary for reliable physical and emotional well-being. No drug can cure an illness – unless the mechanisms of body and mind are functioning in symbiotic alignment. (378)

In 1942 George Miley, a clinical professor at Hahnemann Hospital and College of Medicine, reported 103 cases of acute infections at Hahnemann Hospital in Philadelphia. Such conditions included sepsis, sinusitis, wound infections, peritonitis, thrombophlebitis, polio, toxemia of pregnancy. All were treated successfully with UV light therapy. (377)

In his book *The Cure that Time forgot - Ultraviolet Blood Irradiation Therapy* Robert Rowen reports spectacular detailed hopeless cases responding to UV phototherapy. Some of the patients suffered cerebellar artery thrombosis, pneumonia, pulmonary emboli, femoral leg, deep-venous thrombosis, left sided paralysis, and paralysis of the left vocal cord. "Patients responded dramatically, almost instantly, and had a full recovery in several months." (377)

William Campbell Douglass, MD, author of the book *Into the Light* researched a multitude of extremely different cases from Siberia to South Africa, the United States, and Europe. This book includes a multitude of UV light applications not only in the field of medicine, but in technology as well. Somewhat bitter Douglass remarks, "It's unthinkable that the best solution to stopping the world's killer diseases is being ignored, scorned, and rejected."

Here are some of Campbell's remarkable findings:

UV light and critical infections

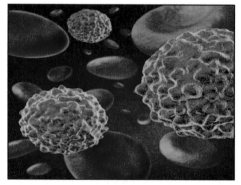

Bacterial endocarditis, an infection of the hearts valves, one of the most dreaded infections observed in medical practice, carries a high mortality rate. Dr. Krishtof and associates treated 250 cases that had undergone prolonged therapy with antibiotics and cortisone with little effect. The patients were given two to three UV light treatments per day. Their hospital stay was significantly shortened. "Predominantly, patients receiving UV-therapy recovered twice as fast from coma." (78)

UV light and blood poisoning
The Ukrainian doctors noted, "a rapid disappearance of intoxication and fever." (78)

UV light and food poisoning
Miley, author in *Archives of Physical Therapy*, Volume 25, June 1944, reports a case of a patient near death from classic botulism neurotoxin. Botulism, a deadly form of food poisoning, causes extreme toxicity and carries a high mortality rate. The patient was unable to swallow or see. The patient was treated with photoluminescence and within 48 hours was able both to swallow and see, and was

completely clear mentally. As Miley said, "There is, to my knowledge, no record in medical science of any other therapy that can produce such an effect on a patient in the last stages of botulism." (78)

UV light and drug intoxication
The Russians have successfully, "treated 128 comatose patients who have been poisoned by organophosphate or had psychotropic drug intoxication." (78)

UV light and pneumonia
Patients with "advanced pneumonia, acute gangrenous appendicitis, multiple pelvic abscesses, and peritonitis have made an undeniable reversal of the threatening situation in 24 to 72 hours." (78)

UV light and coronary arteries
A group of St. Petersburg physicians studied the effect of photoluminescence on 145 patients. These patients suffered from a severe blockage of the coronary arteries after previous heart attack. The doctors chose only patients who had not responded well to conventional drug therapy. (78)

"Significant improvement was registered in 137 of the 145 patients treated with UV light therapy. Pain was quickly relieved and analgesics were often discontinued. The dosage of heart medications, such as beta-blocking agents, was reduced in most patients and the attacks of angina were less frequent than conventionally treated patients." (78)

UV light and thrombosis
Dutkevich and associates reported that 10.3 percent of surgical cases in their series developed some degree of thrombophlebitis or thrombosis after surgery. "Not a single case developed these venous complications once treated with UV light therapy prior to or after surgery." (78)

UV light and military
American as well as Russian troops use UV light Irradiation and radiation for disinfection, medical applications, and for preserving food. (78)

UV light and the American FDA
Ultraviolet irradiation of blood has been approved by the FDA for the treatment of cutaneous T-cell lymphoma. Thus, the method is legal within the context of FDA's definition of legality. It is also legal, from the standpoint of long (over 50 years) and continuous use by physicians in the United States as a commercially viable product before the present FDA was even in existence. (78)

UV light and convalescence
The patients' general state improved almost immediately after the first treatment. Their appetite improved. Hope returned. The patients would often fall into a deep sleep for the first time since their accident.

UV light therapy (photoluminescence) has the remarkable ability to allow the weakened body to make rapid readjustments back to normal biological self-regulation. (78)

UV lights and gout and inflammatory arthritis

Ultraviolet irradiation typically causes the body to eliminate uric acid more rapidly, "suggesting usefulness as a treatment for gout, arthritis, bursitis and other inflammatory conditions of muscles and joints." (78)

UV light and cancer

In 1994 Peter Havasi published his book *Education of Cancer* with countless descriptions of healings promoted through UV light treatments. The following excerpts are taken out of this book:

"In 1967, Robert Olney presented five cases of cancer, which were cured by a combination of techniques, including ultraviolet blood irradiation. He reported the reversal of generalized malignant melanoma in a breast cancer penetrating the chest wall and lung, a highly metastatic colon cancer, thyroid cancer and uterine cancer." (381)

UV light treatments after trauma

"In the field of surgery alone, doctors of the former USSR had used UV therapy in over 100.000 patients. Surgeons Kutushev and Chalenko in St. Petersburg reported that UV therapy cut the number of complications and the necessity of using antibiotics in severe trauma cases by 50 percent. In the past ten years, these two surgeons have successfully treated over 3,000 patients with severe trauma, using UV blood irradiation. Cases ranged from crushed kidneys to extensive bleeding in the chest or abdominal cavities." (381)

UV light with long-term effects

Robert Rowen summarizes his experiences: "Actually, UV blood irradiation therapy may be providing an inactivation of bacteria, a more resistant body, improved circulation, alkalization, etc. It may provide a continuing effect through the secondary emanations of the absorbed ultraviolet rays. Such emissions, which last for many weeks, may account for the observed cumulative effectiveness of the therapy. UV photons, absorbed by hemoglobin, are gradually released over time, continuing the stimulation to the body's physiology." (377)

UV light and uremic pruritus

In 1977 researchers studied the effect of ultraviolet phototherapy on severely persistent pruritus in 18 adult patients on hemodialysis. "Nine out of ten patients treated with UV light reported a distinct decrease in pruritus. The response to phototherapy was unaffected by the presence of secondary hyperparathyroidism." Researchers concluded, "Ultraviolet phototherapy is a safe, convenient, inexpensive and effective treatment for uremic pruritus." (382)

UV light and hepatitis

A study was done in 2015 on nine patients with hepatitis C infection. They received 15 UVBI treatments over the course of 22 weeks. The researchers concluded at the end of the study: "UVBI was safe and had a beneficial effect in the treatment of hepatitis C infection. This device should be studied for use against psoriasis and infectious diseases that have few treatment options." (383)

UV light and chronic kidney disease

A study was published in 2017. Researchers examined different treatments for chronic kidney disease-associated pruritus, amongst them were Ultraviolet-B (UVB) light therapy, gamma-linolenic acid (GLA), thalidomide, turmeric, nicotinamide, sericin cream, pentoxifylline, tacrolimus cream, and ergocalciferol. "Of these treatments, UVB light therapy, and GLA have shown the most promise for treating the chronic kidney disease pruritus. " (384)

Bone marrow cancer in remission after 9 days of Blu Room treatments

In 1990 Nikki Bertone was diagnosed with Multiple Myeloma (bone marrow cancer). She was on a strict regime with chemotherapy and other medication for 5 to 6 years. Eventually her skin turned grey. In January 2016 the cancer came back. On June 1st 2016 she started chemotherapy anew. In October 2016 she chose to add the Blu Room UV light therapy. After nine days of three visits per day, her skin pigment improved, her life energies restored and the mobility regained. Blood work done before and after Blu Room treatment showed dramatic results. The cancer markers were back to normal. (386)

Blu Room users have reported improvements in a wide range of health conditions.

A sampling of data reports: beneficial experiences with anxiety, depression, thyroid disorder, stroke, PTSD/Trauma disorder, osteoporosis, MS, astigmatism, high cholesterol, breast cancer, cancer of the pancreas, ADHS syndrome, joint inflammation, allergies, autism, cerebral palsy, chronic fatigue syndrome, Crohn's disease, diabetes, and many more.

Blu Room users enjoy a wide range of wellbeing.

They report multifaceted happy improvements in the quality of their life. They report more perseverance, higher jumping power, more self-confidence, increased mental presence in negotiations, fulfilled new parenthood, school improvements, and brilliant ideas for the diploma thesis. Some are just so happy, they attract their dream partner. Some accessed a wider field of potentialities and gained new strategic decisions from that. Children dare to register for science competitions. One woman said, "I am now much more confident than ever before. I can accept myself as a valuable woman and demand a fair price for my services."

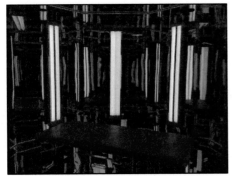

Source: Centro Holistico, San Piero in Bagno (FC), Italy

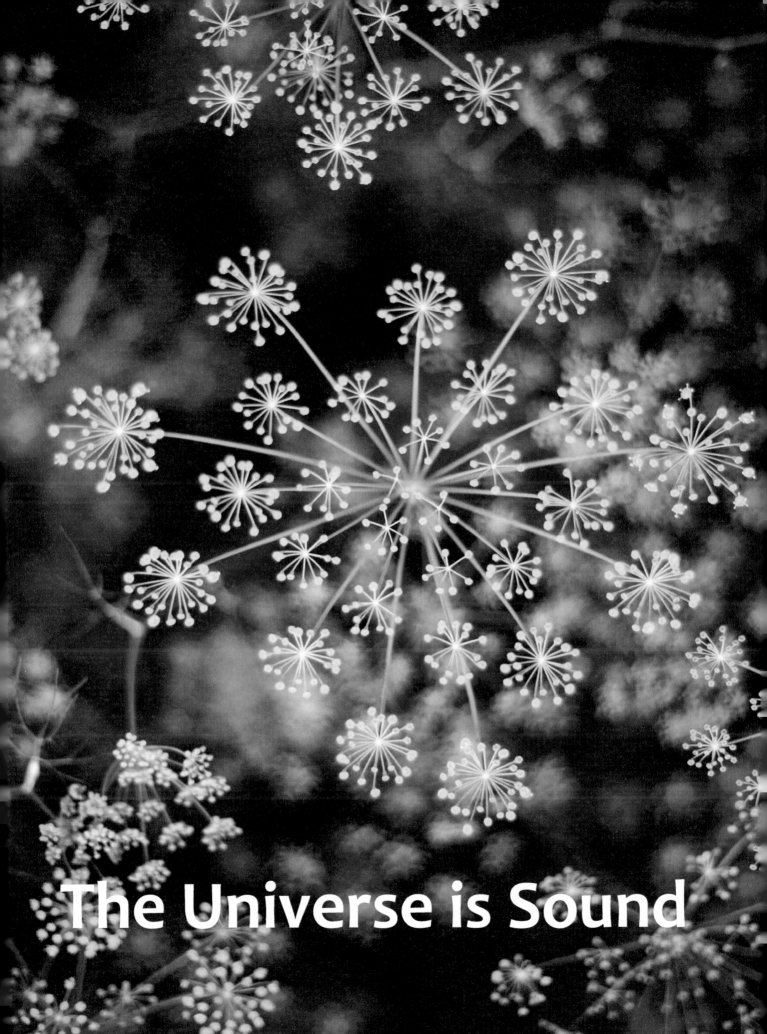

The Universe is Sound

Chapter Five

The Universe is Sound

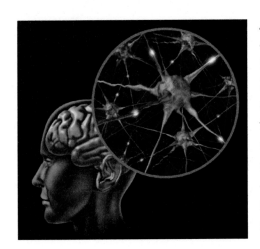

At the root of all our thoughts, emotions, and behaviors is the communication between the neurons in our brain. The average human brain contains about 100 billion neurons, interconnected by trillions of connections, called synapses. Largely, each connection transmits about one signal per second. This is hard to imagine. Some specialized connections even send up to 1,000 signals per second. Vibrant, vast and, complex neural networks – the backbone of the brain's processing capabilities – are constantly attentive. The combination of millions of neurons simultaneously sending signals produces an enormous amount of electrical activity in the brain.

All electrical activity of the brain is commonly called a brainwave pattern, because of its cyclic, "wave-like" nature. Our brainwaves change according to what we're doing and feeling. The brainwaves of a sleeping person are vastly different than the brainwaves of someone wide awake. (387)

An electroencephalogram (EEG) measures and records the brain's activity. Special sensors called electrodes are attached to the head. They're connected by wires to a computer. The computer records the brain's electrical activity on the screen. The electrical impulses in an EEG recording look like wavy lines with peaks and valleys.

Brainwaves

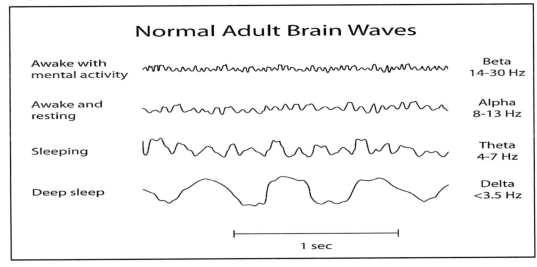

Source: www.integrativelifesolutions.com

The descriptions that follow are only vague descriptions. In reality brainwaves are far more complex. They reflect different aspects when they occur in different locations in the brain. Brain wave frequency is measured in cycles per second or Hertz (Hz). The amplitude, or size and strength of the wave are also measured. Gamma brain waves are the fastest and smallest waves. Delta waves are the slowest and largest. Mind frequency patterns naturally vary throughout day and night depending on how mentally engaged and active a person is.

Five wave patterns define different states of consciousness:
- Beta   – normal waking consciousness
- Alpha – relaxation, dissolved in thought
- Theta – relaxation, meditation
- Delta – deep sleep
- Gamma – mental peak performance

In 1942, the German psychiatrist Hans Berger, the inventor of the EEG discovered alpha and beta brainwaves.

Beta wave
14 – 30 Hz

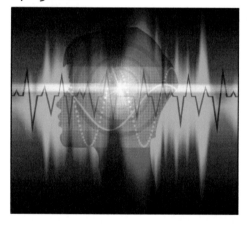

Beta brainwaves dominate the normal active state of consciousness. Beta is often associated with busy, active, or anxious thinking. Beta is present in critical thinking, writing, reading, watching, and social interactions. Higher levels of beta are related to anxiety, stress, separation, and misery. The highest beta frequencies are associated with high levels of arousal.

At the lower end of the beta scale, we are able to produce brain stimulations to trigger positive benefits such as improved learning ability, increased physical energy, and general higher awareness and efficiency. (388)

Alpha wave
8 – 13 Hz
In the early 1960s and 1970s, alpha waves drew much attention due to the application of biofeedback. Biofeedback is a technique to learn to control the body's functions such as the heart rate. An alpha state is the preferred brainwave for achieving this.

Beta represents activation, alpha represents non-activation. This frequency range bridges the gap between our conscious thinking and subconscious mind. In general, the alpha wave is prominent in a person who is awake but relaxed with eyes closed.

Alpha is the resting state for the brain. In alpha sensory inputs are minimized and the mind is generally clear of unwanted thoughts. This is a receptive learning state of mind. This state is related to focused attention and intuition. In a state of joy and wellbeing, alpha is generally present. In alpha, it is easier to change and reprogram the mind to influence health in general.

Theta wave
4 – 7 Hz

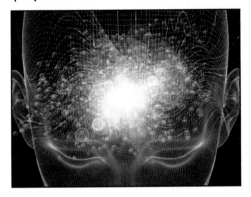

This particular frequency range is involved in twilight daydreaming and sleep. Theta brainwaves frequently occur in sleep or in deep meditation. They act as our gateway to deep learning and comprehensive memory. In theta, our senses are withdrawn from the external world and focused on signals originating from within or respectively the DNA's capability for hypercommunication. (388)

Theta meditational music is said to be capable of promoting "super learning," enhanced creativity, cultivation of ideas, and deep relaxation.

Dr. Thomas Budzynski, one of the world's foremost authorities on biofeedback, affirms that theta waves can induce "a sensation of detached relaxation." The Theta state induces behavioral changes, as well as reprogramming negative beliefs. This in turn, allows a living organism to perform self-healing. "Repair orders and reprogramming go directly into the subconscious, where they are accepted as truths and can have uplifting effects." (389)

Delta wave
0,5 – 3,5 HZ
Delta waves are generated in deepest meditation and in dreamless sleep. Delta waves suspend external awareness and are the source of empathy. This state triggers healings of the body and mind. Certain frequencies in the delta zone provoke the release of Human Growth Hormone (HGH), as well as DHEA and melatonin. (390) According to researchers, "women have been shown to have more delta wave activity, and this is true for most mammal species. This discrepancy does not become apparent until early adulthood (in the 30's or 40's in humans), with men showing greater age-related reductions in delta wave activity than women." (391) Delta waves have also been observed in the deepest states of Zen meditation. (392)

Gamma wave
30 – 70 Hz
Gamma brainwaves have low and virtually unnoticeable amplitude, yet they are the fastest frequency. They originate in the thalamus and traverse to the front of the brain before returning to the thalamus. Due to their fast frequency they can be detected in nearly every part of the brain. With regular production, these brainwaves can help reduce stress, anxiety, and depression, while

improving happiness. (393) According to a popular theory, gamma waves may be implicated in creating a unity of conscious perception, universal love, and altruism.

Gamma waves relate to simultaneous processing of information from different brain areas and have been associated with higher states of conscious perception. A greater presence of Gamma relates to an expanded consciousness and spiritual emergence. Peak performers often have more gamma waves than others. (388)

Healthy rhythm is healthy life

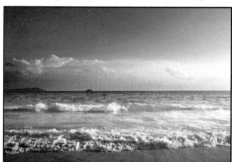

Watching the ocean waves roll in and out, changing the sands surface, riding the breezes, and reflecting the sun's beauty is pure harmony in a healthy rhythm. Mind and body can heal naturally, when in a state of relaxed brain frequencies of alpha, theta, and delta brain waves. The goal of slowing the brain wave frequency is to help master the mind by being attentive to current health and life issues instead of just being at the mercy of past programming from childhood.

Our brainwave profile and our daily experience of the world are inseparable. When our brainwaves are out of balance – out of sync – there will be corresponding problems in our emotional or neuro-physical health. Research has identified brainwave patterns associated with all sorts of emotional and neurological conditions. (394)

"If you want to find the secrets of the universe, think in terms of energy, frequency, and vibration." Nikola Tesla

Healing frequencies – healing sounds

The universe in itself is a gigantic symphony of sound. Each living entity represents a unique underlying numeric property or an exclusive sound. All things are frequency and energy. This endorses the overall harmony of the universe. Everything in the universe is vibrating in tune with all particles contained in it, regardless of size, sex, age, creed, distances, or other peculiarities.

The sound OM

OM represents all time, past, present, and future. It is beyond time itself. OM represents the eternal oneness of all that is. It is the ultimate goal to become unified in body, mind, and spirit. (395)

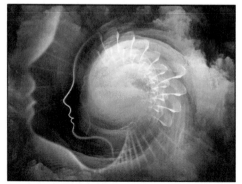

OM is the primordial sound according to Vedic philosophy from which the whole universe was created. It is a sacred sound in Hinduism, Buddhism, Jainism, and Sikhism. The Upanishads are full of references: "The Imperishable is OM. Whatever is visible, whatever is cognizable, and whatever can be sensed, whatever can be comprehended under the single term of creation. All this is OM." (395)

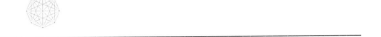

Everything in the universe is pulsating and vibrating – nothing is ever standing still. The Ancient Indian Rishis called 7.83 Hz the frequency of OM. Hertz is the term modern experts use for defining frequency.

The earth has its own frequency wave which is acknowledged by NASA. It was named after the German scientist Winfried Otto Schumann in 1952, "even though Nikola Tesla was the first known person to mention this frequency in 1907." (396)

The 7.83 Hz Schumann Resonance is the bridge resonance between the meditative theta (4-7 Hz) and the deeply relaxed alpha state (8-13 Hz). This "In Between" allows increased ability for harnessing the data acquired in deep levels of the human mind back into a normal relaxed state.

8Hz is said to be the frequency of the double helix in the process of DNA replication, enabling mitosis to occur. A form of body temperature superconductivity is evident in this process. (397)

432 Hz is the frequency of deep harmony
Taking 8Hz as our starting point on a musical scale and working upwards by five octaves we reach a frequency of 256Hz. On this scale the note A has a frequency of 432 Hz.

Verdi's 'A'
According to music theory, A=432 Hz is mathematically consistent with the universe. This is known as Verdi's 'A' – named after Giuseppe Verdi, a famous Italian composer. This tuning to 432 Hz was unanimously approved at the Congress of Italian musicians in 1881 and recommended by the physicists Joseph Sauveur and Felix Savart as well as by the Italian scientist Bartolomeo Grassi Landi. (398). In 1953 in London the worldwide reference frequency was amended to 440 Hz. (399)

There is a global controversy concerning the precise definition for A. The Boston Symphony Orchestra supports A having a frequency of 441 Hz. The New York Philharmonic supports A having a frequency of 442 Hz. In continental Europe, the symphony orchestras support A having a frequency of 443 Hz. (400)

Mozart, Verdi, and Richard Strauss insisted that their music were played in 432 Hz. Many musicians from all nations such as Luciano Pavarotti, Placido Domingo, John Lennon, Birgit Nilsson, Joan Sutherland, Montserrat Caballe to name a few, came forward to change this again to 432 Hz. Some of the early works of Bob Marley (i.e. Three Little Birds) were recorded on instruments tuned to the 432 Hz scale.

Music in 432 Hz is experienced as relaxing and healing; it opens the heart and connects heaven and earth with nothing and everything.

Sound images show the molecular variation at 440 Hz and 432 Hz. (401)

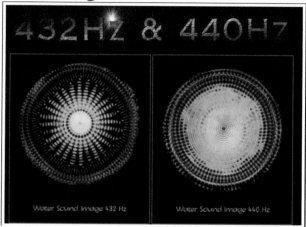

Source: https://www.ideapod.com

Einstein and the harmony of the universe

As a boy Einstein did poorly in school. Music was an outlet for his emotions. At 5, he began violin lessons but soon found the drills so trying that he threw a chair at his teacher, who ran out of the house in tears. At 13, he discovered Mozart's sonatas. (402)

Einstein once said that while Beethoven created his music, Mozart's "was so pure that it seemed to have been ever-present in the universe, waiting to be discovered by its master." Einstein believed much the same of physics that beyond observations and theory lay the music of the spheres -- which he wrote revealed a "pre-established harmony" exhibiting stunning symmetries.

Einstein often turned to the simple beauty of Mozart's music for inspiration. "Whenever he felt that he had come to the end of the road or was in a difficult situation in his work, he would take refuge in music," recalled his older son, Hans Albert. "That would usually resolve all his difficulties." In the end, Einstein felt that in his own field he had, "like Mozart, succeeded in unraveling the complexity of the universe." (403)

Solfeggio frequencies

The Solfeggio frequencies were known to various ancient cultures and have been specifically used by these civilizations for the alleviation and cure of physical and mental illnesses. Even the early Catholic Church was aware of the Solfeggio frequencies and their effects and used them for the composition of many hymns, such as the Gregorian monk chants.

According to Professor Willi Apel, the origin of the ancient Solfeggio scale can be traced back to a medieval hymn to John the Baptist. The hymn has this peculiarity that the first six lines of the music commenced respectively on the first six successive notes of the scale, and thus the first syllable of each line was sung to a note one degree higher that the first syllable of the line that preceded it. Because the music held mathematic resonance, the original frequencies were capable of spiritually inspiring mankind to be more "godkind." (404)

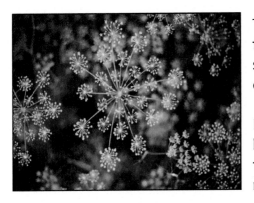

The Solfeggio frequencies are mystical and were once forbidden frequencies even though it was believed that they might support the healing mind and body. The Solfeggio frequencies do not appear in our common twelve-tone system.

In the mid-1970's Dr. Joseph Puleo, a physician and America's leading herbalist, deciphered the pattern used to unfold the frequencies. He applied the Pythagorean method of numeral reduction. It is now called the digital root.

The digital root is a simple reduction method, used to turn big numbers into single digits numbers. The values of all digits in the number are added up. If the number still contains more than one digit after the first addition, the process is repeated. Here's an example: 456 can be reduced to 4+5+6 = 15, and subsequently reduced to 1+5=6. So the number 456 eventually reduces to the single digit 6.

All Solfeggio frequencies sum up to 3 – 6 – 9.

174 Hz	Association	digit sum 3
285 Hz	Universal knowledge	digit sum 6
396 Hz	Liberating from guilt and fear	digit sum 9
417 Hz	Undoing situations and facilitating change	digit sum 3
528 Hz	Transformation and DNA repair	digit sum 6
639 Hz	Harmonic connections/relationships	digit sum 9
741 Hz	Awakening Intuition	digit sum 3
852 Hz	Returning to Divine Order	digit sum 6
963 Hz	God Man, God Woman	digit sum 9

The 3, 6, and 9 are the fundamental root vibrations of the Solfeggio frequencies.

In modern molecular biology 528 Hz is used to repair the frequency of damaged DNA strands. In order to reprogram DNA, the cell membrane must first be opened to allow access to the DNA. It is said, "the frequencies of the Solfeggio incite the opening of the cell for new imprints on the DNA." (405)

Masaru Emoto, Doctor of Alternative Medicine captured water's 'expressions.' He developed a technique using a very powerful microscope in a very cold room along with high-speed photography. Under these circumstances he photographed newly formed crystals of frozen water samples, once they were exposed to frequencies.

Emoto discovered that crystals formed in frozen water reveal changes when specific, concentrated thoughts or frequencies are directed toward them. He found that water from clear springs and water that has been exposed to loving words showed brilliant, complex, and colorful snowflake patterns. In contrast, polluted water, or water exposed to negative thoughts, revealed incomplete forms and asymmetrical patterns with dull colors. (406)

Impressive sound images of the effect of 6 Solfeggio tones in form of water crystals (407)

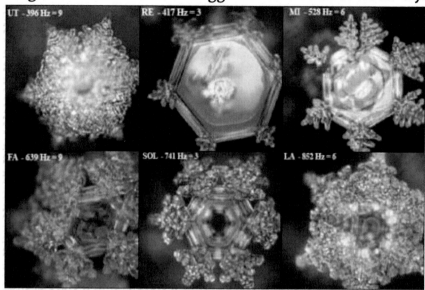

Source: www.galacticfacets.com

Sound patterns of Solfeggio's frequencies can be found: ttp://www.mamuriel.de/Ch_Klaenge.htm

The song of the planet Earth

All matter vibrates at specific levels and everything has its own melody. The musical nature of nuclear matter from atoms to galaxies is being recognized by science. Sound waves cannot travel through the vacuum of space. Electromagnetic waves can. These electromagnetic waves can be recorded by devices called spectrographs with many of the world's most powerful telescopes.

The original frequencies are much too high for humans or even dogs to hear. These electromagnetic waves are converted into sound waves. They were reduced 1.75 trillion times. This allows us to listen to many parts of the universe for the first time. "We can hear the song of a comet, the chimes of stars being born or dying, the choir of a quasar eating the heart of a galaxy, and much more." (408)

Oct. 1, 2012: A NASA spacecraft has just beamed back a beautiful song sung by our own planet. "It's called a chorus," explains Craig Kletzing of the University of Iowa. "This is one of the clearest examples we've ever heard." (409)

It's a planet of sound! Sound starts with just a simple vibration. It's at the heart of everything.

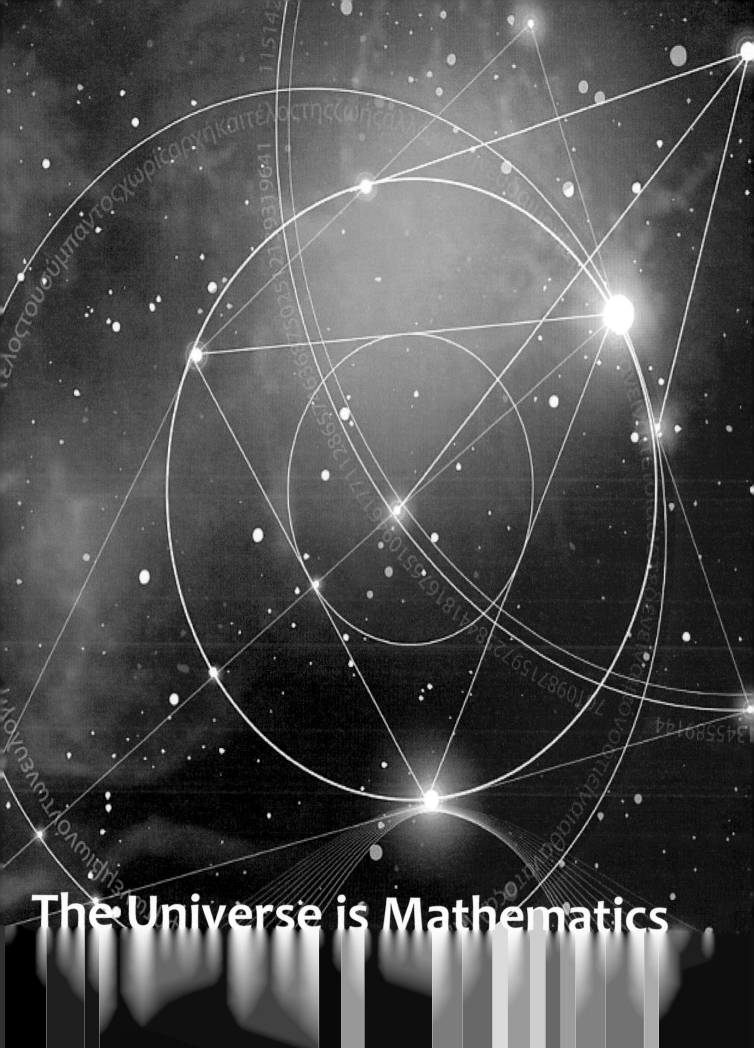

The Universe is Mathematics

Chapter Six

The Universe is Mathematics

Nikola Tesla, the unique genius and father of the alternating current, once said, "If you only knew the magnificence of the 3, 6, and 9, then you would hold the key to the universe."

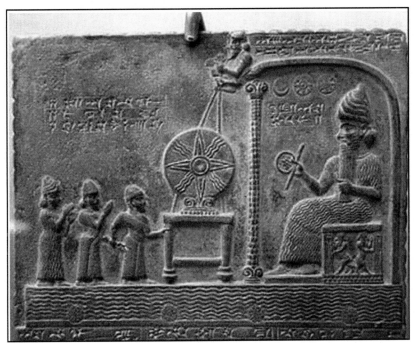

The Tablet of Shamash – Ancient Sumer
Source: wikipedia.org

In the ancient Sanskrit texts of the Vedas, we find the evidence of dividing a circle into 360 parts.

Twelve spokes, one wheel, navels three.
Who can comprehend this?
On it are placed together
three hundred and sixty like pegs.
They shake not in the least.

Dirghatamas, Rigveda 1.164.48 (410)

Based on what is commonly believed today the Sumerians of ancient Mesopotamia were the first people to divide the circle into 360 equal parts at around 3000 BC. The Sumerians understood astronomy, light, medicine, and higher mathematics. They also had excellent engineering skills, well developed agriculture, and knowledge of the wheel. Where did this knowledge come from? Was hypercommunication their natural way to access information? This tablet may answer some questions. (411)

The circle and the number 3-6-9

For thousands and thousands of years mathematicians have solved difficult calculations with the help of digital roots. It is recorded that the ancient Sumer and Babylonians and the Indian Vedic math used digit roots. Pythagoras formalized them in 530BC. A digital root is the single digit to which long numbers break down via the addition of all the digits.

In dividing a circle into 360° equal parts we always see the following a pattern of 180°, 90°, 45°, 22.5°, 11.25, 5.625°, 2.8125°, etc. The resulting angles always reduces to nine. For example, the digit root of 2.8125 = 18, digit sum of 18 = 9

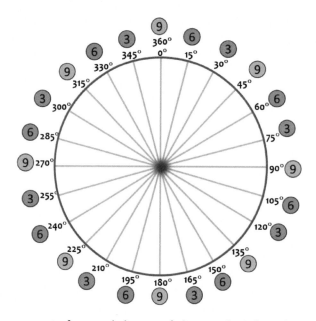

Let us divide a clock in 24 segments for each hour of day and night. Then write in every segment the number of seconds per hour. Adding all seconds, it sums up to 766,800. Each digit root of every segment adds up to nine and the digit root of all seconds together make 9. The nine shows up in the center. A vortex is being created. Time is overcome. (410)

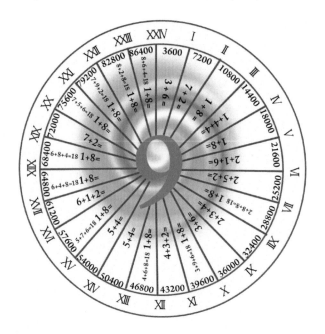

Nine is the number of perfection and divine symmetry

Is there a divine code embedded in our numeric system? Generally speaking, a code can be either:

- a collection of laws or regulations relating to a specific activity or subject
- a rule for transmitting a secret message from one symbolic form into another with little or no loss of information
- a computer code, or
- a set of instructions in a program.

According to the ancient Vedas

- Nine consists of the All-Powerful 3 x 3.
- Nine is three times the triad.
- Nine is completion, fulfillment, wholeness, beginning and end.
- Nine is a heavenly and angelic number and symbolizes earthly paradise.
- Nine is an indestructible number.

Nine is the number of the circumference, its division into 90 degrees and 360 degrees for the whole perimeter. It is symbolized by the figure of the two triangles. This in turn is a symbol of the principle of male and female, fire and water, mountain and cave. (412)

Nine represents achievement and completion. There are 9 months in pregnancy, 9 initiations during our advancing from a lower stage to a higher stage.

Pythagoras states: Nine is the limit of the numbers, because all other numbers exist in it and return to it. (413)

The sum of all digits excluding nine is 36: 1+2+3+4+5+6+7+8= 36, and 3+6=9. Paradoxically, nine plus any digit returns to the same digit: 9+7= 16, and 1+6=7. So nine literally equals all digits (36) and nothing (0). Nine models all things potentially and no things materially. (414)

The symbol of the Nine is the spiral. Spirals represent the unity of thought and being, life and death. It is space, time material and immaterial at the same time. It is an ancient symbol from many

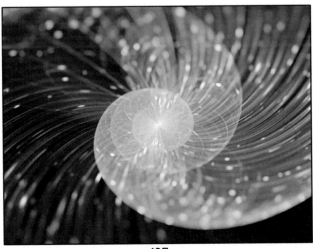

cultures, as a principle of the macrocosm and microcosm.

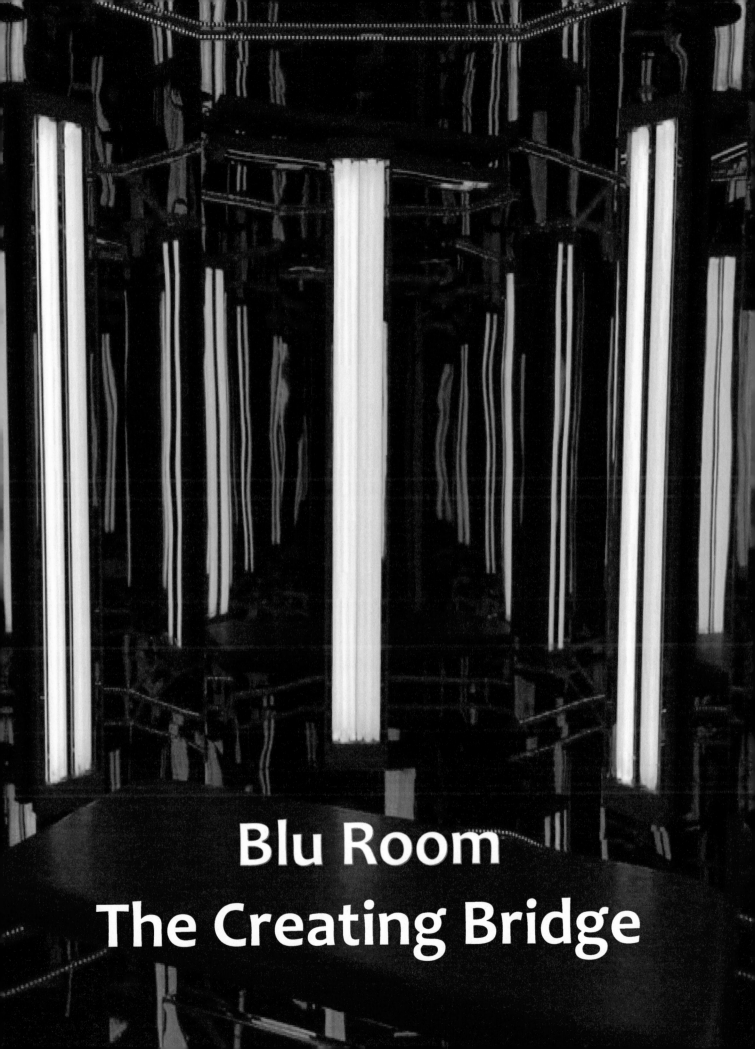

Blu Room
The Creating Bridge

Chapter Seven

Blu Room - The Creating Bridge

Blu Room and its Architecture

The Blu Room is an octagon-shaped room that bridges ancient and futuristic.

The octagon is a significant geometric shape and symbol throughout human history symbolizing: (415)

- Regeneration
- Totality
- Infinity
- Rebirth
- Transition

The Tower of the Winds in Athens, Greece is the oldest known octagonal building and was built in approximately 300 B.C. It served as a marble horologium or "timepiece."

The builders of octagonal buildings were mostly kings and emperors of particular stature such as Frederick II. He built the great Castel del Monte. Frederick had powerful enemies at this time. He was frequently at war with the papacy.

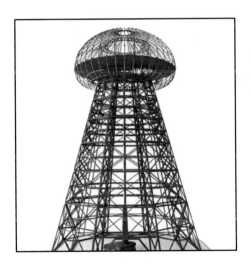

In 1901, Nikola Tesla built this wooden 57 meters high octagonal building, called Wardenclyffe Tower in Shoreham, New York. He erected this tower, "as the first broadcasting system in the world, and transmitting electrical energy without wires [freely] to the globe using the Ionosphere." (416) No limitations and energy loss due to cable networks.

The octagon "represents the ultimate balance between matter and invisible forces, the fixed male and mutable female; total balance between material and spiritual, heart and mind. It is both the inhalation and the exhalation of the breath of creation." (410)

The Greek philosopher Pythagoras believed the "eightness" of the Octagon was the "Embracer of Harmonies" and linked it to safety, constancy and everything that was balanced in the universe.

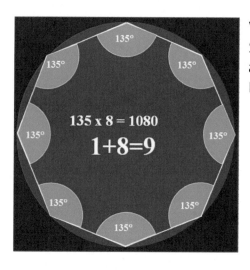

When looking at the octagon from the perspective of the Sumerians, the number nine comes forth. The sum of each angle leads to nine and the digit sum of all angles make up NINE. Completion – no beginning no end.

$135 \times 8 = 1080$

$1+8=9$

Blu Room and the magic mirror

The architecture of the Blu Room is an octagon. It has 72-inch long UVB lamps installed on each wall of the octagon and on the ceiling.

The nine lamps used in the Blu Room emit medical narrowband UVB radiation. The person lies on a therapeutic bed in the middle of the Blu Room. Thus, every single cell in the body receives intensive, selective UVB irradiation with all its life supporting effects. This allows a high efficiency without side effects.

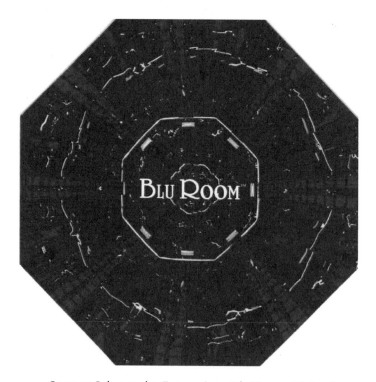

Source: Salamander Enterprises, Blu Room Kägiswil

The octagon of the Blu Room is shielded with a glistening mirror-like material from side to side, from bottom to ceiling, from each corner to all other corners. Some users call it a cathedral.

Blu Room and reflection

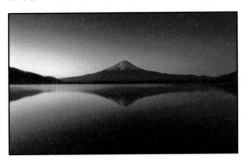

One of the earliest accounts of light reflection originates from the ancient Greek mathematician Euclid. He authored a series of experiments around 300 BC. He had a good understanding of how light is reflected. A millennium and a half later the Arab scientist Alhazen specialized on optics. He authored more than 100 works on optics, astronomy, and mathematics. He is regarded as one of the greatest scientists, although his name is scarcely known. Alhazen was the first scientist to describe the refraction and the dispersion of light into its component colors, although hundreds of years later Isaac Newton was credited for this. In Ahazen's *Book on Optics* he established his theories of vision, light and color, as well as his research in catoptrics (study of optical systems using mirrors) and dioptrics (the study of the reflection and refraction of light). (417) He was the first to divine a law describing exactly what happens to a light ray when it strikes a smooth surface and then bounces off. (418)

The law of reflection states that when light falls upon a plane surface and is reflected, the angle of incidence is equal to the angle of reflection. This law is used when the incidence ray, the reflected ray, and the normal all fall upon a plane area of incidence.

In the diagram, the ray of light approaching the mirror is the incident ray. The ray of light that leaves

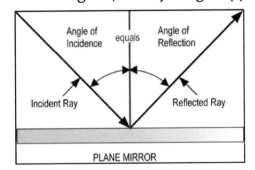

the mirror is the reflected ray. At the point of incidence where the ray strikes the mirror, a line is drawn perpendicular to the surface of the mirror. This line is called the normal line or equals. The normal line divides the angle between the incident ray and the reflected ray into two equal angles. The angle between the incident ray and the normal is known as the angle of incidence. The angle between the reflected ray and the normal is known as the angle of reflection. (419)

Source: www.student-tutor.org

In wave theory light waves spread out

Light acts either as a wave or as a particle. Examining the reflecting qualities of light, different theories have emerged. According to wave-based theories, the light waves spread out from the source in all directions. Once they hit the mirror, they are reflected at an angle determined by the angle at which the light arrives. The reflection process inverts each wave back-to-front. This is the reason why a reverse image is observed. (419)

In particle theory light arrives as a stream

According to particle theory, light arrives at the mirror in the form of a stream of tiny particles, called photons. These micro tiny particles hit the surface and bounce back. Yet the particles are so small and travel very closely together that they bounce off from different points. "Their order is reversed by the reflection process, producing a mirror image." The electrons in the atoms of the blackened side of the mirror absorb the photons in light. "In turn, these atoms emit new photons, causing a reflection." The photons coming out of a mirror are not the same ones that went into it. (419)

The result of reflection is the same, regardless of the light acting as a wave or particles.

The amount of light reflected by an object, and how it is reflected, is highly dependent upon the degree of smoothness or texture of the surface. (419)

Blu Room and vibration

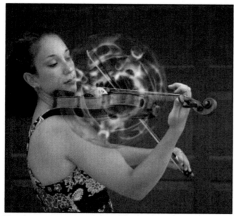

Source: www.energyfanatics.com

Sound causes a system to oscillate, to vibrate. Sound is a special form of transmission of information. Sound is at the core of all things. It has stimulation effects on mind and matter. Listening to music can stimulate the imagination in many directions; it may arouse memories of past experiences or blast into future potentialities. The Blu Room is pure vibration.

The Law of Vibration, a law of nature, states that nothing rests; everything moves; everything vibrates. The lower the vibration, the slower it is; the higher vibration, the faster it is. (420)

The Law of Vibration applies to all things; sound, colors, the cells in our body, the food we eat and even our emotions and thoughts. (421) It serves as the foundation for the Law of Attraction.

The article *Frequency & the Law of Vibration* states that the difference between the manifestations of physical, mental, spiritual, and emotional wellbeing is the result from different levels of vibrating energy or frequencies. (422)

Scientists claim that these frequencies control the molecules in our body. In 1974, Dr. Colin W.F. and colleagues from the Oxford University discovered, "that frequencies of vibrating energy are roughly one hundred times more efficient in relaying information within a biological system than physical signals, such as hormones, neurotransmitters and other growth factors." (71)

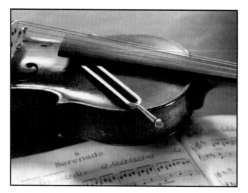

Applying this principle of resonance to Blu Room experiences, self-healing becomes clear. Once the person lies comfortably in the middle of the room, the sound of the music begins to enchant. The UV lights are turned on and create a radiant, dazzling atmosphere. UVB light hits the skin, enters through the upper layer and accelerates vibrational pulses into the inner core of the DNA. Anxiety and stress give way to deep relaxation.

The principle of resonance in physics states that when two frequencies are brought together, the lower will always rise to meet the higher. In tuning a piano, a tuning fork is struck, and then brought close to the piano string that carries that same musical tone. The string then raises its vibration automatically and attunes itself to the same rate at which the fork is vibrating. This is exactly what happens in the Blu Room. Frequencies of fear, grief, and loneliness are changed into the prevailing higher frequencies of happiness, relaxing, regenerating, and rejuvenating.

A very powerful structured coherent photonic field supports the activities in both the DNA and the mitochondria. This is a state of absolute harmony. The cells are deeply relaxed to their inner core. In this state, repair and regeneration begin. Every second 10 million cells die and 10 million new cells are generated. In a three-minute Blu Room session 180 billion cells are newly generated, imprinted with the innate harmony of a stress-free DNA.

From each millimeter of this awesome geometry, soft UV radiation radiates into the center, reflecting itself and in doing so it envelops the person in a creative vortex of light, detachment, and oneness. Time ceases to exist.

Nikola Tesla – Pioneer in healing with frequency vibration
"The day Science begins to study non-physical phenomena, it will make more progress in one decade, than in all previous centuries of its existence!" – Nikola Tesla

In 1891, the inventor Nikola Tesla designed a power supply for his "System of Electric Lighting." It is

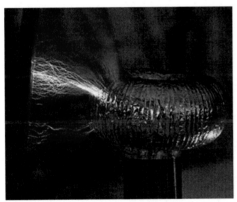

known as the Tesla coil. Tesla used this resonant transformer circuit to conduct many innovative experiments in electrical lighting, phosphorescence, X-ray generation, high frequency alternating current phenomena, the transmission of electrical energy without wires, and electrotherapy. (423)

A whole branch of medicine was founded on the healing effects of certain Tesla coil frequencies (High Frequency Air-Core Resonant Transformer). Tesla understood the therapeutic value of frequency vibrations.

Source: www.teslasociety.com

It is reported that, "patients just sitting in the vicinity of vibrations from a device like [a variation of the Tesla coil] experienced relief from rheumatism and other painful conditions. It was even considered to be a cure for certain types of paralysis. Such radiations increased the supply of blood to an area with a warming effect (diathermy). They enhanced the oxygenation and nutritive value of the blood, increased various secretions, and accelerated the elimination of waste products in the blood. All this promotes healing." (424)

Blu Room and its atmosphere

The word "atmosphere" derives from ancient Greek and Sanskrit.

ATMOS meaning steam
SPHERE   meaning a ball

Viktor Schauberger, an Austrian scientist and inventor from the last century came from a family of foresters and spent much time in nature. In his observation of the natural world he came to recognize a subtle, yet powerful ordering force, that he called "Creative Intelligence, the divine creative intention in action." (425)

Viktor Schauberger regarded the atmosphere as the vital amniotic fluid that surrounds the Earth. The Earth floats in this atmosphere, nourishing it and protecting it from the potentially destructive forces of the cosmos. (426)

The Earth breathes like a living being, and in pulsing it derives its basic feminine energies in accordance to its rotation and in response to the energy received from the sun.

The creative principle of the pulsating DNA oscillates and vibrates in rhythmic cycles, contracting and expanding anew. Just as the DNA rhythmically contracts during light intake and expands during light output, so do all the other small and large systems, organisms or their components, in fact the entire world of phenomena. This pulsation is found everywhere in nature. It prevails by the principle of contraction and expansion, of inhaling and exhaling, attraction and repulsion, involution and evolution, etc.

The pulsating field in the Blu Room is like this vital amniotic fluid in which the person floats in a calming oneness of sound, light, vibration, frequency and solitariness. He is nourished and protected from destructive forces. A new constitution unfolds.

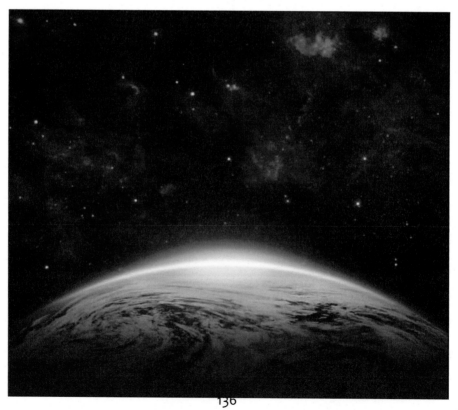

The Blu Room in Action

Light repairs

A cell, even when damaged by 99 percent, can regenerate itself completely, once it is irradiated with weak ultraviolet light. Experiments have shown that this is also a proven fact in higher organisms, including humans. (427)

A 2013 study takes a look at *Sunlight and Vitamin D as a global perspective for health*. Researchers confirm that "during exposure to sunlight radiation with wavelengths of 290–315 nm penetrates into the skin and is absorbed by proteins, DNA and RNA as well as 7-dehydrocholesterol. It is thus able to protect DNA and RNA from photo damage." (97)

Cancer is a loss of coherent light

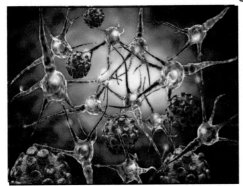

In his later years Prof. Dr. Popp was convinced he found a key to cancer-treatment. He identified important aspects of two rather closely named chemical substances. "Benzo(a)pyrene, a polycyclic hydrocarbon which is considered the most harmful carcinogen for humans, whereas its twin, who differs from it only by a tiny deviation of the molecular composition, benzo(e)pyrene is harmless." He irradiated both molecules with ultraviolet light, to find out why two almost identical molecules differ so completely.

"He discovered that benzo(a)pyrene (the cancer producing molecule) absorbed the UV light, then re-emitted it at a completely different frequency — it was a light "scrambler." The benzo(e)pyrene (harmless to humans), allowed the UV light to pass through it unaltered." Popp was puzzled by this difference, and continued to experiment with UV light and other compounds. After some investigations Popp could see that carcinogenic substances absorb ultraviolet light and change or destroy its frequency. (429)

If cancer-causing chemicals could alter the body's biophoton emissions, then it might be that other substances could reintroduce better communication. Popp wondered whether certain plant extracts could change the character of the biophoton emissions to enhance cell to cell communication. He began experimenting with a number of non-toxic substances claimed to be successful in treating cancer. The only effective substance he measured was mistletoe. (429)

Popp found out that cancer patients lack healthy coherent rhythms. (430) The coherence is the key to health and disease. Health is a state of perfect subatomic communication. Biophotons establish this communication. Disease is a condition in which this communication is disrupted or broken down.

Cell to cell communication in the Blu Room

How cells "talk" to each other

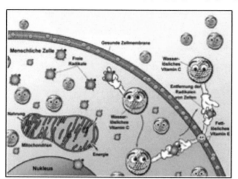

When you get a cut or a scratch on your skin, the injured cells signal the surrounding healthy cells to begin reproducing copies of healthy cells to fill in and mend the opening. When the skin is back to normal, a signal is sent to the cells to tell them to stop reproducing.

How is it possible that tens of thousands of different molecules recognize their respective target in the body? How can the immune system tackle antibody specific foreign invaders and render them harmless? Who is telling the proteins where to dock on different partner proteins or be injected into specific nucleic acids to control gene expression? A mechanical, physical explanation seems a bit far-fetched when considering that per second in only one cell hundreds of thousands of responses are calculated and executed.

There is much evidence that the biophoton radiation of living cells not only covers more than just the range of visible light. It acts as a radio transmitter for cells. Each molecule radiates a unique electromagnetic field, which can "read the field of the complementary molecule." Sayer Ji, the author of an article published March 2017 in *The Event Chronicle* writes, "Biophotons are used by the cells to communicate for energy or informational transfer that is several orders faster than chemical diffusion." (431) The molecules move according to this rhythm. Biophotons provide the code; vitamin D hormones execute the message.

Veljko Veljković and Irena Cosic argued that molecular interactions are electrical in nature and travel distances, which are enormous compared to the size of molecules. Cosic later introduced the concept of dynamic electromagnetic field interactions. This states that "molecules recognize their respective goals by electromagnetic resonance." The molecules emit electromagnetic waves of certain frequencies, enabling them to see and hear, "because these electromagnetic waves can take both the form of photons and phonons." They can influence each other via long distance and attract each other passionately and irresistibly. In each cell hundreds of thousands of chemical reactions take place per second. "This can only happen if the reacting molecules are affected by a respective photon. Once a photon triggers the response, it returns to the field to be used for further reactions." (432)

"Everything is energy and that is all there is to it. Match the frequency to the reality you want and you cannot help but achieve that reality. There can be no other way. This is not philosophy. This is physics." (432)

The miracle in the microtubules

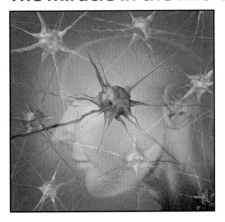

Microtubules are a component of the cytoskeleton, which is present in all cells of all domains of life. They can grow as long as 50 micrometers and are highly dynamic. The outer diameter of a microtubule is about 24 nm while the inner diameter is about 12 nm. They are involved in maintaining the structure of the cell. Traditionally microtubules are regarded as the cell's 'bone-like' scaffolding.

In their pioneering work, Dr. Stuart Hameroff (433), professor of anesthesiology at the University of Arizona and Sir Roger Penrose, English mathematician and theoretical physicist describe the brain as a quantum computer whose main architecture consists of cytoskeleton microtubules. These are encountered in each individual neuron cell of the brain structures. (434) Microtubules and other cytoskeletal structures play a communicative role. Microtubule lattices can interact with neighboring tubulins to represent, propagate and process information as in molecular-level 'cellular automata' computing systems." (4)

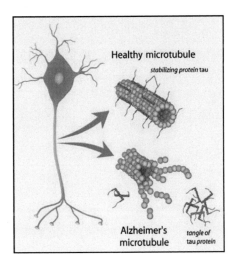

Healthy microtubule

stabilizing protein tau

Alzheimer's microtubule

tangle of tau protein

If one examines a neuron, one discovers numerous hollow tubes that surround the axon. These microtubules previously hold a kind of scaffolding to support the nerve fiber. At second glance these microtubules might well prove to be the structural elements of our consciousness.

The microtubules are predetermined for quantum effects. Their properties are the crystalline lattice structure, the hollow inner core, the organizational function within the cells and the ability to process information. According to the findings of the researchers their size is perfectly suited for transmitting photons in the UV range. (434)

In order to move the biophotons through the micro tubes, they are sent to the synapses of the neuron to move it to the next neuron. So, microtubules provide the wiring system for coherent light in the brain and the rest of the body. Hameroff speaks of a network designed like the internet of the organism. It enables the exchange of information of quanta between the brain and the rest of the body. All cells of the body have the same perception simultaneously.

If the system is disturbed, it does not function properly. Degenerations or even disintegration of microtubules is the result. The activity of biophotons is interrupted. The disturbed cell-to-cell communication causes disorder, stress, and failure to detect, block and cover up.

The British Mathematician Roger Penrose also arrives at the same conclusion that "consciousness and the interaction of different levels of consciousness can be explained by the wave function collapse in the microtubules of the brain. The thin microtubules tunnels that run through the brain represent in their entirety a bio-computer, based on quantum effects. In the tiny cavities called microtubule quantum coherences are absolutely conceivable." (435)These are the chords of quantum oscillations, similar to a finely tuned orchestra.

Microtubules are essential for the stimulation of self-healing. They transfer order and empower the cells through the nervous system in a biophoton rich field. This encourages order, or even recovery. The Blu Room is a powerful order imaging system, due to its architecture, the mild UV rays, the reflection, and the harmonizing sounds.

Dr. Kerstin Bortfeldt runs the first European Blu Room in Germany. She reports, "Experiences in Blu Room indicate that the stimulation of self-healing properties are typical recurring reactions when we come into contact with a greater dimension. I personally see this as a crucial key to the enormous Blu Room effects on self-healing. We know so far, that disturbing thoughts are dimmed in the Blu Room and self-healing brain areas are stimulated. This activates the interdimensional communication in the microtubules increasingly. Strong vibrations are perceived by Blu Room users exactly within the affected body regions when addressing imbalances, blockages, or traumas. This is in my view nothing more than quantum coherence in the microtubules. In this case it is triggered by ultraviolet blue frequencies and reflection. " (436)

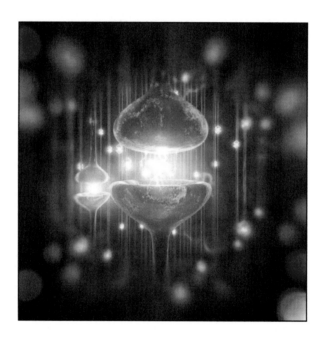

Blu Room and the sunshine vitamin

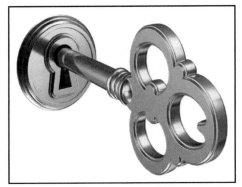

Vitamin D is unique. It is so essential to life, that the body has the ability to generate it thru the skin once exposed to sunlight. General life or our biological body depends on a constant presence of vitamin D. The sun's UVB light strikes the skin, and the body synthesizes vitamin D3 in its richest form. Skin derived vitamin D is biologically inert. The hydroxylation process begins in the liver, prepares for the next enzymatic conversion step in the kidney until the biologically active form of vitamin D the calcitriol, 1,25(OH)2D3 is available. Calcitriol increases the level of calcium in the blood by increasing the uptake of calcium from the intestines into the blood.

A vitamin D receptor is present in most tissues and cells in the body. (437) Vitamin D hormones use these receptor for docking and performing further activities. Evidence indicates that the synthesis of vitamin D from sun exposure is regulated by a feedback loop that prevents toxicity. Why is that? This generation of vitamin D is solely based on the individual's present situation and of course DNA input. The vitamin D is unique for this one person; it is frequency specific to the innate DNA. It is endogenous. No additional enzymes and synthesis are needed. No conversion losses, no transportation difficulties, no cognitive disorders, and no occupied receptor sites ensue. As soon as the first rays touch the skin, messengers clear the transport channels and stimulate the receptor sites. Vitamin D has the right of way, even into the most precious DNA.

The vitamin D hormones produced in a short time and in large numbers in the Blu Room conditions swirl like a spiral throughout the body. This is fundamental, because virtually every cell needs vitamin D for controlling intercellular processes. Whether the body is healthy or develops chronic diseases, it depends on an adequate supply of active vitamin D3.

Vitamin D3 is essential for

- the brain (e.g. depression),
- the immune system (e.g. infection protection, auto-immune protection),
- the cardiovascular system (i.e. blood pressure regulation),
- cancer (i.e. suppressed tumor growth),
- bones and muscles (i.e. strengthening),
- the pancreas (i.e. insulin regulation),
- mental development and longevity,
- and on stem cell growth

Vitamin D generated in the Blu Room plays a vital role. Vitamin D as hormone grants good health, creativity, youthfulness, and physical and spiritual renewal. Vitamin D opens doors into a realm of long forgotten potentials.

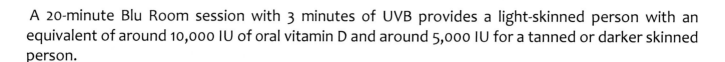

A 20-minute Blu Room session with 3 minutes of UVB provides a light-skinned person with an equivalent of around 10,000 IU of oral vitamin D and around 5,000 IU for a tanned or darker skinned person.

A 20-minute Blu Room session with 6 minutes of UVB provides a light-skinned person with an equivalent of around 20,000 IU of oral vitamin D and around 10,000 IU for a tanned or darker skinned person.

A 20-minute Blu Room session with 9 minutes of UVB provides a light-skinned person with an equivalent of around 30,000 IU of oral vitamin D and around 15,000 IU for a tanned or darker skinned person.

Blu Room and structured water

The philosopher and astronomer Thales of Miletus (640-546 BC.) describes water as the only real element from which all other bodies are created. He believes that it is the fundamental substance of the universe.

Pioneers such as Albert Szent-Gyorgyi knew that water's role in biology is fundamental. Szent-Gyorgyi states: "Life is water dancing to the tune of solids." (438) He is commonly regarded as the father of modern biochemistry. He was rewarded with the Nobel Prize for discovering vitamin C.

Dr. Gerald Pollack, a professor of bioengineering at the University of Washington showed, that electromagnetic energy, whether in the form of ultraviolet (UV) wavelengths or infrared wavelengths change the molecular structure of water into a self-ordering structure. The molecules reorganize and build a charged and ordered zone. Pollack calls this the fourth phase of water, the EZ zone (exclusion zone). It is also called the "In-Between-Zone."

Water is an essential part of life on Earth. Water is special not only because it covers over 70 percent of the earth's surface, but also because it is the only known substance that can exist in gaseous, liquid, and solid phases within a relatively narrow range. The exclusion zone is exactly the mediating zone in between zones. It is this zone, where water is not solid anymore, yet not quite liquid. This zone is a bridge-medium which responds to UV light 270-310 nanometers radiation, as Pollack discovered. Water becomes structured and oxygenated. Pollack calls this water H_3O_2. Structured water appears to be stable; it has no resistance like rainwater. It holds its structure and the energy even if stagnant for some time. The more structured a water becomes, the more potential it has for enhancing hydration and cell to cell communication. (439)

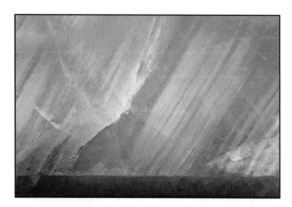

"Glacial ice carries the same structured order, since it is permanently exposed to UVB light. A lot of people have known that this water is really good for your health," Dr. Pollack says. (439)

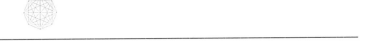

Based on Dr. Pollack's theories Blu Room irradiated is water structured and oxygenated. This water stays stable in its high oxygenation for quite a long time. After a Blu Room session, every person is provided with this water.

Blu Room and deep relaxation

> "It is the way inwards to our own center. The inner stillness invites any intuition and creativity to come forth."
> Steve Jobs (440)

According to the Oxford dictionary, "relaxation is when the body and mind are free from tension and anxiety." Relaxation is the emotional state of low tension, in which there is an absence of highly energetic emotions. Fear, insecurity, anger, anxiety, or even being madly in love are a few of these active emotional states. Relaxation reduces stress signals. Stress is the leading cause of mental and physical problems. Stress activates the sympathetic nervous system into a fight-or-flight response mode. Chronic stress leads to harmful effects on the body.

While in this UV-induced unpolarized field, the body as a whole organism and every individual cell can relax. No polarities, neither fight nor flight, neither rat race nor boredom, neither victim nor tyrant.

Deep relaxation can be dramatically effective in relieving symptoms such as inflammation, anxiety, and muscle tension. It can be a lifesaver when dealing with physical, emotional, and psychological stress. Combined with thoughts of clear intent, it can vastly improve our ability to perform at optimal levels even when taking on some of life's greatest challenges.

By relieving tension, circulation is improved and healing accelerated. Used before surgery, one needs less anesthesia, has less postoperative pain, leaves the hospital sooner, and recovers with minimal complications.

Studies done in a state of deep relaxation show effects on
- Sport performance, stress reduction and gerontologic research. (University of Illinois),
- Drug addiction and following de-dependency (San Francisco State University),
- pain reduction with lasting effects (Massachusetts General Hospital, Boston),
- accelerated learning and stimulation on psychosomatic problems. (University of Iowa),
- a decrease of depression related symptoms (University of Giessen, Germany),
- the access of sub consciousness (Verein FOCUS, Vienna, Austria),
- treating adolescent depression (Dr. Jacques Puichaud, UPEA, La Rochelle, France),
- accelerated learning, effects on intelligence (University of Essen, Germany),
- treating insomnia. (Dr. Bernard Ferracci, psychiatrist, Paris, France),
- relief from chronic headaches and migraines (Department of Internal Medicine at the U.S. Air Force Medical Center)
- psychosomatic skin disorders,

- providing mental clarity,
- improving sleeping patterns (for sleep preparation and sleep duration),
- allowing for better physical detoxification by the liver,
- stimulating immunology functions,
- enhancing creativity,
- calming patients before and after surgery,
- accessing altered states of consciousness.
- Average increases of the beta-endorphin and serotonin levels were registered. (441)

A study by the Menninger Foundation found that people who accessed theta brain waves had "new and authentic ideas, not primarily by deduction but springing from intuition from unconscious sources." (442)

Further evidence that theta waves promote creativity and innovation comes from Dr. Roman Chrucky, Medical Director of the North Jersey Developmental Center. Dr. Chrucky has been experimenting with brainwave entrainment tools in his practice for some time, and notes from his research that, "a lot of people spontaneously told me that they've felt much more creative." His personal experience backs this up, "I've found that using the theta frequency I get that kind of response as well, increased creativity." (442)

Once you are in the Blu Room, a cocoon of ultraviolet blue light embraces you, you close your eyes, you are hardly aware of the music, and your breathing calms down. Your body is in an alpha state simply by closing your eyes. The vitamin D floods your body with hormones of wellbeing and regeneration. One of the first things you may notice is a quiet body response and restored energy resources. On top of this, a light degree of trance is induced which helps you to process knowledge from a deeper level while the body regenerates. The Blu Room provides a solitariness and comforting safety that allows you to give yourself permission to relax, to let go, and to trust the innate guidance while in this deeply relaxed and open state.

Soon you may reach a theta-wave induced twilight state. Vivid imagery, intuition, and information beyond our normal conscious awareness can be accessed. During deep relaxation, the mental state you enter is similar to that of a young curious child.

Dr. Thomas Budzynski, one of the world's foremost authorities on biofeedback, states that theta-waves can induce "a sensation of detached relaxation." (443) Theta state changes behavior as well as reprogramming negative beliefs. This in turn allows a living organism to accomplish self-healing. "Repair orders and reprogramming go directly into the subconscious, where they are accepted as truths and can henceforth have a positive effect." (389)

One of the main benefits of using deep relaxation is that you are able to exercise control over the thoughts that enter your mind. You can choose which thoughts to keep and which ones to abandon. You begin to grasp the power you hold to change your life for the better.

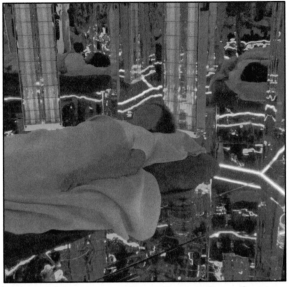

The aim in the Blu Room is to "let go" of the day and float completely in the present. The Blu Room works without any conscious effort. You will soon find yourself drifting into a peaceful, calm and relaxed state within just a few minutes. It is delightfully simple, blissful and beneficial. Just let your mind go and enjoy feeling relaxed and happy, while the innate hidden intelligence guides your body to heal and realign the DNA.

The Blu Room is a solitary cocoon of ease. It's a neutral zone where the mind is present in the moment, attached to nothing and totally centered.

The architecture, the mirrored surfaces, all frequencies, and all sounds meet in the center, while being constantly reflected. Your own DNA and every cell respond. You experience the magic of NINE.

Nine is the all and nothing
Without beginning without end
Neither black nor white
Neither good nor bad
Neither right nor wrong
Neither plus nor minus.
Neither cold nor warm

The NINE is completion. Changes can take place. It is your choice.

The Blu Room works by itself, there is no need to believe, no need to analyze, and no need to understand. Not everything has to be proven. Some things can simply be experienced.

Users have reported a wide range of personal beneficial experiences, including:
- Deep relaxation
- Faster healing processes
- Relief from physical pain
- Relief from mental stress & anxiety
- Improved health and well-being
- Deepened focus
- Increased creativity
- Greater self-awareness
- Significant increases in Vitamin D3

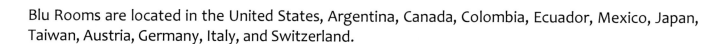

Blu Rooms are located in the United States, Argentina, Canada, Colombia, Ecuador, Mexico, Japan, Taiwan, Austria, Germany, Italy, and Switzerland.

Locations are available at www.bluroom.com/pages/locations.aspx. Over 50,000 sessions have been provided as of October 2017.

Blu Room is the future in medicine and personal well-being.
Blu Room affects you physically, mentally and spiritually.
Blu Room puts you back in charge of your life.

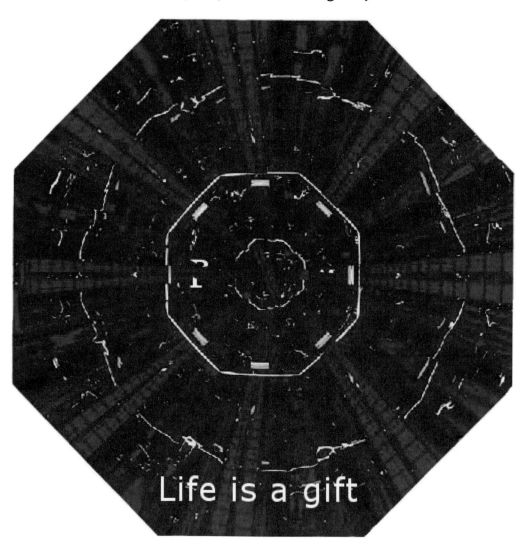

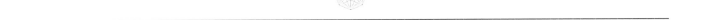

Interview with JZ Knight, the inventor

JZ Knight invented the Blu Room in 2015. She is a member/manager of Blu Room Enterprises, LLC. Below is a transcript of her interview with Mark Alyn in the Late Night Health radio show on December 12, 2016 (lightly edited for readability).

Ultraviolet Light Therapy - The Blu Room experience

Mark: We are talking to JZ Knight, who invented the Blu Room based on the work of Nikola Tesla. Welcome JZ. What is the Blu Room experience?

JZ: I am so honored to be on your show. The Blu Room is a physical room in the shape of an octagon. It has a UVB balanced light in each octagon parcel. UVB light with medical frequency. The walls are covered with stainless steel, so it is a mirrored room experience, with a bed in there. One enters for a 20 minute session. Within the 20 minute session is a graduation of three to nine minutes where the lights are on and then a rest period after the lights go off.

Mark: That means I won't get a tan or I won't get cancer?

JZ: Exactly, but you feel terrific. In designing the octagon, I used the mathematics from Nikola Tesla. With the mathematics in the construction of the octagon, the center equals nine. According to Nikola Tesla, nine is the greatest number and nothing. It is everything and nothing. It is the most etheric number we have. When you lay on the bed, the effect of the mathematics of the room with UVB lights on, with mirror reflection, it looks like eternity. Within that certain area, right where nine exists, we lay there in an atmosphere. All of this creates an atmosphere. I call it that because it is where we have a meeting of all that goes into this room in sacred geometry, mathematics, and UVB light. Within this atmosphere we can become completely rested. For example, in just three minutes with the UVB lights on, one gets about 10,000 IU vitamin D.

Mark: Which we need. We need the UVB to make vitamin D. We have a shortage of vitamin D. We have a shortage in our diets as well as a deficit in our bodies.

JZ: This is a chronic health issue. If you go six minutes, you get 20,000 IU, nine minutes is 30,000 IU. That is for lighter skin; less for darker skin. When we lay there, there is a confluent and wonderful things will happen. The greatest vitamin D you can get is thru the ultraviolet spectrum of sunlight. When your skin is exposed like in photosynthesis, the skin takes in the UVB light, causing the cells in the body to produce vitamin D, which I call the God hormone. Vitamin D creates a whole chain reaction within the body. We are rather sort of like plants. We come up as seedlings but we don't get enough light so we don't flourish fully in our health and our vitality. In the Blu Room, we get that. So just imagine most people are walking around as feeble seedlings that have not really reached their health capacity, their vitality capacity. In the room we get this without being exposed to the dangerous frequencies of the sunlight, getting cancer, getting a tan. People think a tan is cool, but it is really breaking down the skin processes, we get wrinkles and faded skin.

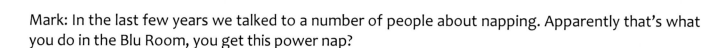

Mark: In the last few years we talked to a number of people about napping. Apparently that's what you do in the Blu Room, you get this power nap?

JZ: Yes, you get this power nap. You lay under these lights in the atmosphere and what happens in this configuration is a form of stasis. This is the best term I can find - stasis. We reach physically and spiritually a harmony, a stasis point. This stasis point actually means that if we take the old concept of good and bad and everything is in a yin yang concept, if your mind is going back and forth, your body is always in confusion and it too is going back and forth. The body follows the mind. The genes as a genetic code follow our mind. So through the most miraculous concept of stasis, what happens in the room is that those positive and negative thoughts cease. We have this unity of everything in harmony. We just lay there and – because it is so restful not having this internal battle with one's mind of good and bad thoughts – a deep relaxation occurs. At the same time our body is now through photosynthesis producing vitamin D throughout the body creating this whole cascade of effects.

Mark: It seems to me it is a chance to rejuvenate.

JZ: Not only rejuvenate – how about kick start health? In over 50,000 user sessions so far, individuals have experienced deeper relaxation and healing processes. Our list of maladies, injuries and diseases is extensive. We don't claim that this going to heal everything. All we do say is that one gets exposed to vitamin D. Just imagine a seedling is coming up a little bit, someone takes the cover off and sunlight shines and in one day it has grown immensely. We are like that when we come out of the Blu Room. But the spiritual and consciousness concept of the room can come into play too. Simply bring your mind to stasis and allow the process of rejuvenation to work. People may go in stressed out, yet they come out of it absolutely without stress and anxiety. It relieves physical pain, any pain anywhere. We have it on every level. Also, we just finished a small test group of eleven PTSD patients, active and inactive veterans, with really severe cases. We did this small test for about 60 days. It changed nearly everything for them.

Mark: I want to be in one.

JZ: Please come. I would love you and Carol to come and experience it. You would love this room, because it is a divinely inspired room. Our reports of people coming in with an enormous array of maladies from cancer to pain, every joint, every part, every organ in the body and a whole list of diseases. One thing we can say about the Blu Room other than the fact that we have stasis is we have a lessening – even a removal – of pain. It goes away for about three days.

Mark: In going into the Blu Room I am thinking of energy healing, because there is energy obviously in the UV light. I had energy healing. It knocks me out, I just fall asleep. When I wake up, I feel refreshed, I feel great, I don't want to leave. Is that kind of the feeling?

JZ: Yes, but we are not only getting a physical turnaround in our body. We really cannot heal the body unless we approach the mind, unless we approach a person's thought processes. Consciousness is also energy, they are inextricably combined. You cannot have consciousness

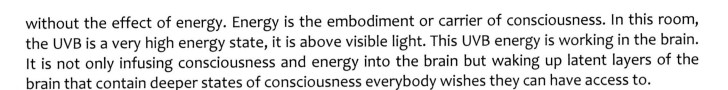

without the effect of energy. Energy is the embodiment or carrier of consciousness. In this room, the UVB is a very high energy state, it is above visible light. This UVB energy is working in the brain. It is not only infusing consciousness and energy into the brain but waking up latent layers of the brain that contain deeper states of consciousness everybody wishes they can have access to.

Mark: It would seem to me, being in that room with what you have just said, that your creativity goes up and your pain goes down. Your love of life increases because you feel good.

JZ: You feel good. Stress goes away. No anxiety. Deep relaxation. In other words, it is a reset.

Mark: JZ how did the idea come to you, to create this little slice of heaven?

JZ: Actually, it did come from heaven. It's been a desire of mine for a very long time to bring back such an atmosphere based on my experience in another conscious realm. I finally brought it back and built this realm in a room. We are now working in the Blu Room with stem cells, and by the way, with food too. I opened the Blu Room up after I put it through a test done by a very nervous doctor. He allowed it to come in his clinic and he was so overjoyed just by the relief of pain and stress and anxiety or reduction in blood pressure. Skin effects were going away, multiple sclerosis effects were coming down. He was so blown away. He became my business partner and our oversight physician. But when we encounter reflective mathematical geometry and UVB light in a certain specific criteria setting we experience stasis. All of this has to be together. Yes, it is a divinely inspired room. It does much more than just giving us vitamin D. But if that's all that it did, relieving depression, if all that it did was to cure PTSD, if all that it did was to bring us to a point of happiness – no confusion in our brain – without medication! There are no side effects to the Blu Room. The only side effect is just really happy people.

Mark: Thank you so much. Hope to hear from you soon.

Questions and answers with Dr. Matthew Martinez
February 2017 in Switzerland.

Dr. Matthew Martinez practices as a physician and chiropractor. He is a member/manager of Blu Room Enterprises, LLC. Dr. Matt also owns two clinics that provide Blu Room services – Absolute Health Clinic in Olympia, WA and The Tree of Life Center in Riobamba, Ecuador.

Why do you call this room an atmosphere?
The architecture, the sound, the frequency, and color generate the brilliant highly tuned atmosphere of the Blu Room. Yet everybody brings their own atmosphere. The atmosphere in the room is generated by you. When you enter that Blu Room, you are present. When your own atmosphere is weak and you are feeling sick, your atmosphere is immediately uplifted. When two frequencies are brought together, the lower will always rise to meet the higher. This is the principle behind the tuning fork. Now you are free to create. What do you want to be? Do you want to be healthy or sick? Most people want to be healthy.

I talk a lot about children, for they are closer to God than adults. They have no blocks. What is the child's atmosphere? Happiness! They wake up in the morning and say, what is going on today, everything is possible. I love my boys. When they come every morning into my room, Mikey throws the door open and says, "I am back." And then he is playing, doing something, building, experiencing. When Mikey goes to the Blu Room, he runs into my office, runs into the Blu Room, closes the door and is ready. His atmosphere is whatever he needs it to be, pure joy.

What is the meaning of music in the Blu Room?

Music plays such a big role. I am Latin, music is rhythm. When my family gets together we dance, we have music, everyone in my family gets an instrument and we make music. Whether you are good at it or not.

Music is life. When you open the window you hear the machinery of mankind, but in the backdrop it sings, the universe sings, the universe is music. Everything has a harmonic frequency. Music is so important in every culture. When we hear a song and it is an important song to us, it doesn't matter what the song is, it pulls emotions, it pulls energy, and it pulls memory. It'll either make you cry or be happy or you know you just don't like it. Music is so powerful. When we get down to what music is, it is always frequency, vibration. And the frequency and vibration can be either healing or detrimental. Animals communicate. How do they communicate? Sound. Yet it sounds like music. Whales sing. It is beautiful. The vibration of that music travels. Music in the Blu Room is an added frequency. We know 432 Hz music is extremely healing for the body. This is music designed to heal the DNA. That is why we have music in the Blu Room. It is one more added goblet to help the body heal. Music also relaxes and calms down, wiping away daily pressure.

Why do some people heal better than others?

It is because of the neuro-immune system response. They are able to have a response that is quicker, clearer and stronger without any interference. Children don't know they cannot heal. They heal very fast. And children have more stem cells than adults. They love to go outside, love to eat, and love to be happy. Most adults work indoors, they are busy, don't eat well, don't exercise, and definitely don't spend time in the sun. Why? "I don't want to have wrinkles, don't want to damage my skin, don't have time" – or even fear of sunspots.

We were not designed to be sick or weak, we are designed to be healthy and have all the benefits of a healthy body. We are the responsible part for poisoning the earth, poisoning our food, our water, our air. This is because of greed. For so many people, money is more important than health, more important than love, more important than relationships, but money will never heal.

What are your experiences with multiple sclerosis?

Complete reversal with Blu Room without stem cells – no side effect, no surgery. When a person had an autoimmune disease for a long time, his stem cells are important. The disease is very aggressive. MS is a common disease. It is a direct result of long continuing vitamin D deficiency. There is a very specific geographic distribution of this disease around the world. A significantly

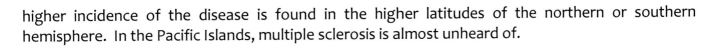

higher incidence of the disease is found in the higher latitudes of the northern or southern hemisphere. In the Pacific Islands, multiple sclerosis is almost unheard of.

How much vitamin D do we need?
Without vitamin D your cells cannot function properly. They can't, we know this. Any doctor who is out there telling you don't need vitamin D is wrong. You have to have it every day. And more and more we understand that you need a daily minimum of 5.000 to 10.000 IU to function physiologically.

What happens if you don't get vitamin D? How many different diseases are associated with vitamin D deficiency? Everything from schizophrenia, depression, skin problems, nervous system problems, digestion problems, cancer, muscle wasting, it goes on and on and on. I could fill pages – at least 1500 different diseases are noted.

Do you have experiences with headaches or migraines and the Blu Room?
With the Blu room we have great success with migraines. Very often headaches are caused by a vitamin D deficiency or the inability of the body to assimilate vitamin supplements.

Don't underestimate the constant bombardment of radiation we presently live in. Wi-Fi is everywhere. We are surrounded by radio frequencies. It is the first time in our history that the earth is bombarded with theses rays. Where are the long-term studies for this? Where are the long-term studies on these mobile phones? What I recommend to you is to take a break, turn off Wi-Fi at night. Try to not use them for about 8-10 hours a day. Who remembers the time when we didn't have them? Did we survive? A little prediction: we will see more brain tumors in the coming years than we have ever seen. Mobile phones don't work in the Blu Room. I designed it that way. Your mind is totally free; at rest.

What do you think about antibiotics? They kill bacteria too.
You know about the germ theory? Louis Pasteur. The environment. If the germ theory were true, we would all be dead. We are all exposed to bacteria and viruses daily. Why are we not dead? Our physiology is much better than what science gives us credit for. Ask anyone says that antibiotics saved us all, how did we survive before we had the antibiotics? New research is coming out that antibiotics were never that good and are only important when somebody is about to die. But we started giving antibiotics for every infection. The body is now resistant to many antibiotics. So we are going back to all those age-old medicines from thousands of years ago. Vitamin D or sunshine plays an important role.

What does the Blu Room do for people with depression?
I have seen this many times when people come into my office with massive depressions, often they are suicidal. I work with a lot of soldiers who suffer under post-traumatic stress disorder and there is no cure. The soldiers had very traumatic experiences. They are very depressed, have relationship problems, sleep problems, digestion problems. All they think of is getting rid of this life. I know many stories of the Blu Room experiences where these people have completely changed. They are not depressed or sad anymore, they sleep, they have the courage for new relationships, they want

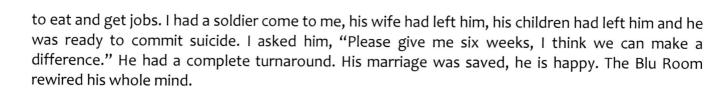

to eat and get jobs. I had a soldier come to me, his wife had left him, his children had left him and he was ready to commit suicide. I asked him, "Please give me six weeks, I think we can make a difference." He had a complete turnaround. His marriage was saved, he is happy. The Blu Room rewired his whole mind.

In what other situations is the Blu Room beneficial?

That is a great question. Many parents are sending their children to us, just to visit the Blu Room. The school approved and the children are more relaxed and less hyperactive. We have several students coming right before they have a difficult exam; they go into the Blu Room, and afterwards head right to the exam. The brain is active. The enhanced cell-to-cell-communication allows a faster comprehension and correct interface of long-term and short-term memory.

We once had the president of a big company come into the Blu Room. His company was in a difficult situation. He had to make far reaching decisions and needed clarity. The Blu Room session cleared his mind and afterwards he could see the greater perspective.

Once a young man came heart broken. His girlfriend has left him. The Blu Room session relieved his grief; he smiled with regained trust when he came out.

I remember a really obese woman came to me. She wanted to lose weight and expected a strong protocol. I advised her to visit Blu Room for four weeks, twice a week – that was all. After these sessions the woman had already lost five pounds and she had regained love for herself. She was happy. If you hate yourself because you feel fat, there is hardly any chance of losing weight and keeping your healthy metabolism upright.

Do I have to believe that the Blu Room is working?

In my clinic in Ecuador I see at least 600 patients a week. Patients come from all over the world. Mostly we have normal diseases like cardiovascular diseases, brain disorders, autoimmune deficiencies or influenzas.

One night at 2 a.m. in the morning, somebody knocked at my gate. A mother and father were standing there, carrying their 8-year old boy. "Doc, you have to help us. Our son has been kicked out of the hospital with liver cirrhosis cancer to die at home." I am a father, so I asked them to come in. On the examination table the fearful eyes of the boy looked at me, he had a bloated belly, yellow eyes and face. It looked very bad. The mother and father were very sad. I had a moment with the boy by myself and asked him, "Do you want to live?" All he said was, "I want to play." Since it was already sunrise, my own little boys came running to see where Papa is. The little boy's eyes lit up. Hope, to be able to play with these other boys sparked in his veins. We immediately began with the Blu Room sessions and stem cell therapy. The boy is now up and running around my house, playing with my boys.

Hope. Your spirit lives on hope. When we don't have hope, we will die. The little boy had hope. To play again, was all he hoped for. The Blu Room adds to the spirit of hope. (453)

Not everything has to be proven. Some has to be experienced.
Be bold, dare to explore the unknown.

Light, frequency, and sound are the medicine of the future.
Two genius minds, JZ Knight, the inventor and Dr. Matthew Martinez, the co-developer, designed this Blu Room.

The Blu Room is for the newborn and the 109-year-old grandma, for go-getters and lazy-bones, for people on water- and chemotherapy, for pregnant women and nervous fathers, for brilliant inventors and street cleaners, for people of all races and creeds, for the deaf and the blind. The Blu Room is for the stubborn as well as for the smarty, for the young artist and the virtuoso, for the doubting and unshakable, for the dying and mourning, for the politician and money launderer, for the optimist and pessimist, for the country physicians and advocates, for the soldier and the war veteran, for the believer and nonbeliever, for the drunkard and ascetics, for the doubter and fundamentalist, for the hungry and the rich, and for the surgeon and the medicine woman. Light, sound, and frequencies in the Blu Room build bridges and enable the future to be experienced at first hand. The Blu Room is love.

Glossary

Antigen
An antigen is a substance that induces an immune response in the body, specifically the production of antibodies. Antigens may be toxins, foreign proteins, particulates, or organic matter such as bacteria and tissue cells.

Atherosclerosis
Atherosclerosis is the hardening and thickening of the artery walls. It is the most common cause of heart disease, which is the number one killer in America. All arteries, including the aorta, are made up of three layers: the adventitia, the media, and the intima. The intima is the layer that is in direct contact with the blood, whereas the media surrounds the intima and is made up of mostly connective and muscle tissue. The adventitia is the outer-most layer of the arteries.

Biophotons (from the Greek meaning "life" and "light")
Biophotons are photons of light in the ultraviolet and low visible light range that are produced by a biological system. They are non-thermal in origin, and the emission of biophotons is technically a type of bioluminescence, though bioluminescence is generally reserved for higher luminance luciferin/luciferase systems. The term biophoton used in this narrow sense should not be confused with the broader field of bio photonics, which studies the general interaction of light with biological systems.

Biological tissues typically produce an observed radiant emittance in the visible and ultraviolet frequencies ranging from 10–17 to 10–23 W/cm2 (approx. 1-1000 photons/cm2/second). This low level of light has a much weaker intensity than the visible light produced by bioluminescence, but biophotons are detectable above the background of thermal radiation that is emitted by tissues at their normal temperature. (Wikipedia)

Alexander Gurwitsch, who discovered the existence of biophotons, was awarded the Stalin Prize in 1941 for his mitogenic radiation work. Prof. Dr. Popp expanded on his work.

Johanna Budwig (30 September 1908 – 19 May 2003)
She was a German biochemist and author. Budwig was a pharmacist and held doctorate degrees in physics and chemistry. Based on her research on fatty acids she developed a diet that she believed was useful in the treatment of cancer.

While working as a researcher at the German Federal Health Office she noted many cancer drugs being evaluated in the 1950s contained sulphydryl groups. Budwig believed sulphydryl compounds were important to cellular metabolism and cellular respiration. Budwig researched the theory that a low oxygen environment would develop in the absence of sulphydryl groups and/or fatty acid partners that would encourage the proliferation of cancerous cells.

She developed paper chromatography techniques to identify and quantify fatty acids. Budwig used these techniques to compare the fatty acid profiles of sick and healthy individuals. This made her one of the first scientists to consider the health implications of fat consumption, according to Mannion et al. in a 2010 paper in the journal Nutrients. Dr. Budwig was a Nobel Prize nominee. (www.budwig-stiftung.de)

Circadian rhythm
Circadian rhythm is any biological process that displays an endogenous, entrainable oscillation of about 24 hours. These 24-hour rhythms are driven by a circadian clock, and they have been widely observed in plants, animals, fungi, and cyanobacteria.

The term circadian comes from the Latin circa, meaning "around" (or "approximately"), and diēm, meaning "day". The formal study of biological temporal rhythms, such as daily, tidal, weekly, seasonal, and annual rhythms, is called chronobiology. Processes with 24-hour oscillations are more generally called diurnal rhythms; strictly speaking, they should not be called circadian rhythms unless their endogenous nature is confirmed. (www.crystalinks.com/biologicalclock.html)

Although circadian rhythms are endogenous ("built-in", self-sustained), they are adjusted (entrained) to the local environment by external cues called Zeitgebers (from German, "time giver"), which includes light, temperature and redox cycles.

Coherent states
In physics, specifically in quantum mechanics, a coherent state is the specific quantum state of the quantum harmonic oscillator. It is often described as a state which has dynamics most closely resembling the oscillatory behavior of a classical harmonic oscillator. It was the first example of quantum dynamics when Erwin Schrödinger derived it in 1926, while searching for solutions of the Schrödinger equation to satisfy the correspondence principle. The quantum harmonic oscillator and hence, the coherent states,

arise in the quantum theory of a wide range of physical systems. For instance, a coherent state describes the oscillating motion of a particle confined in a quadratic potential well. (reddit PHYSICS)

The coherent state describes a state in a system for which the ground-state wave packet is displaced from the origin of the system. This state can be related to classical solutions by a particle oscillating with an amplitude equivalent to the displacement.

Garjajev, Dr. Pjotr

Russian biophysicist and molecular biologist Pjotr Garjajev and his colleagues at the Russian Academy of Sciences have been carrying out cutting-edge research the nature of DNA. They simply did not believe that 90 percent of our DNA is "Junk DNA." According to Garjajev's studies, DNA is not only the transmitter and receiver of electromagnetic radiation (in the form of energy), but it also absorbs information contained in the radiation and interprets it further. Thus, DNA is an extremely complex interactive optical biochip. (www.rexresearch.com)

Digital roots

Digital roots have been recorded for thousands of years, formalized by Pythagoras in 530 BCE and even earlier in Indian Vedic math. Digital root is the single digit to which long numbers break down via the addition of all the digits. The digital root makes it easy to recognize certain patterns. Secret societies use digital roots to explain hidden truth.

DNA transcription

Transcription is the process by which the information in a strand of DNA is copied into a new molecule of messenger RNA (mRNA). DNA safely and stably stores genetic material in the nuclei of cells as a reference, or template. Meanwhile, mRNA is comparable to a copy from a reference book because it carries the same information as DNA but is not used for long-term storage and can freely exit the nucleus. Although the mRNA contains the same information, it is not an identical copy of the DNA segment, because its sequence is complementary to the DNA template.

Transcription is carried out by an enzyme called RNA polymerase and a number of accessory proteins called transcription factors. Transcription factors can bind to specific DNA sequences called enhancer and promoter sequences in order to recruit RNA polymerase to an appropriate transcription site. Together, the transcription factors and RNA polymerase form a complex called the transcription initiation complex. This complex initiates transcription, and the RNA polymerase begins mRNA synthesis by matching complementary bases to the original DNA strand. The mRNA molecule is elongated and, once the strand is completely synthesized, transcription is terminated. The newly formed mRNA copies of the gene then serve as blueprints for protein synthesis during the process of translation. (www.nature.com)

Einstein, Albert (March 14, 1879 – April 18, 1955)

Einstein was a German-born theoretical physicist. He developed the general theory of relativity, one of the two pillars of modern physics (alongside quantum mechanics). Einstein's work is also known for its influence on the philosophy of science. Einstein is best known in popular culture for his mass–energy equivalence formula $E = mc^2$. He received the 1921 Nobel Prize in Physics "for his services to Theoretical Physics, and especially for his discovery of the law of the photoelectric effect," a pivotal step in the evolution of quantum theory. (Wikipedia)

Near the beginning of his career, Einstein thought that Newtonian mechanics was no longer enough to reconcile the laws of classical mechanics with the laws of the electromagnetic field. This led him to develop his special theory of relativity. He then realized that the principle of relativity could also be extended to gravitational fields, and with his subsequent theory of gravitation in 1916, he published a paper on general relativity. He continued to deal with problems of statistical mechanics and quantum theory which led to his explanations of particle theory and the motion of molecules. He also investigated the thermal properties of light which laid the foundation of the photon theory of light. In 1917, Einstein applied the general theory of relativity to model the large-scale structure of the universe.

He was visiting the United States when Adolf Hitler came to power in 1933 and, being Jewish, he did not go back to Germany where he had been a professor at the Berlin Academy of Sciences. He settled in the United States, becoming an American citizen in 1940. On the eve of World War II, he endorsed a letter to President Franklin D. Roosevelt alerting him to the potential development of "extremely powerful bombs of a new type" and recommending that the US begin similar research. This led to what would become the Manhattan Project. Einstein supported defending the Allied forces but generally denounced the idea of using the newly discovered nuclear fission as a weapon. Later, with the British philosopher Bertrand Russell, Einstein signed the Russell–Einstein Manifesto, which highlighted the danger of nuclear weapons. Einstein was affiliated with the Institute for Advanced Study in Princeton, New Jersey, until his death in 1955.

Einstein published more than 300 scientific papers along with over 150 nonscientific works. On 5 December 2014, universities and archives announced the release of Einstein's papers, comprising more than 30,000 unique documents. (www.curious.astro.cornell.edu/physics)

Emoto, Masuru (July 22, 1943 – October 17, 2014)
Emoto was a Japanese author, researcher, photographer and entrepreneur, who claimed that human consciousness, has an effect on the molecular structure of water. Emoto's conjecture evolved over the years, and his early work explored his belief that water could react to positive thoughts and words, and that polluted water could be cleaned through prayer and positive visualization. (Wikipedia)

Since 1999, Emoto published several volumes of a work entitled Messages from Water, which contain photographs of ice crystals and their accompanying experiments. Emoto's ideas appeared in the movie "What the Bleep Do We Know!?"

Emoto believed that water was a "blueprint for our reality" and that emotional energies and vibrations could change the physical structure of water. Emoto's water crystal experiments consisted of exposing water in glasses to different words, pictures or music, and then freezing and examining the aesthetic properties of the resulting crystals with microscopic photography. Emoto made the claim that water exposed to positive speech and thoughts would result in visually pleasing crystals being formed when that water was frozen. Negative intention would yield ugly frozen crystal formations. (awarenessmag.com)

Euclid of Alexandria
Euclid was a Greek mathematician, often referred to as the "father of geometry." He was active in Alexandria during the reign of Ptolemy I (323–283 BCE). His book Elements is one of the most influential works in the history of mathematics, serving as the main textbook for teaching mathematics (especially geometry) from the time of its publication until the late 19th or early 20th century. In the Elements, Euclid deduced the principles of what is now called Euclidean geometry from a small set of axioms. Euclid also wrote works on perspective, conic sections, spherical geometry, number theory, and rigor. (www.geni.com/people)

FDA - Food and Drug Administration
FDA or USFDA is a federal agency of the United States Department of Health and Human Services, one of the United States federal executive departments. The FDA is responsible for protecting and promoting public health through the control and supervision of food safety, tobacco products, dietary supplements, prescription and over-the-counter pharmaceutical drugs (medications), vaccines, biopharmaceuticals, blood transfusions, medical devices, electromagnetic radiation emitting devices (ERED), cosmetics, animal feed, and veterinary products. (Wikipedia)

The FDA was empowered by the United States Congress to enforce the Federal Food, Drug, and Cosmetic Act, which serves as the primary focus for the Agency. The FDA also enforces other laws, notably Section 361 of the Public Health Service Act and associated regulations, many of which are not directly related to food or drugs. These include regulating lasers, cellular phones, condoms, and control of disease on products ranging from certain household pets to sperm donation for assisted reproduction.

Feynman, Richard Phillips (May 11, 1918 – February 15, 1988)
Feynman was an American theoretical physicist known for his work in the path integral formulation of quantum mechanics, the theory of quantum electrodynamics, and the physics of the super fluidity of super cooled liquid helium, as well as in particle physics for which he proposed the parton model. For his contributions to the development of quantum electrodynamics, Feynman, jointly with Julian Schwinger and Sin-Ichiro Tomonaga, received the Nobel Prize in Physics in 1965. (www.timelineindex.com)

Finsen, Niels Ryberg (1860 – 1904)
Finsen was awarded the Nobel Prize in 1903 "in recognition of his contribution to the treatment of diseases, especially lupus vulgaris, with concentrated light radiation, whereby he has opened a new avenue for medical science."

Finsen developed Pick's disease while in his 20s. In 1903, he described how the disease had influenced his scientific development, "The disease was responsible for my starting investigations on light: I suffered from anemia and tiredness, and since I lived in a house facing the north, I began to believe that I might be helped if I received more sun. I therefore spent as much time as possible in its rays. As an enthusiastic medical man I was of course interested to know what benefit the sun really gave. I considered it from the physiological point of view but got no answer. I drew the conclusion that I was right and the physiology wrong." (Journal of the Royal Society of Medicine)

Fractal
A fractal is a mathematical set that exhibits a repeating pattern displayed at every scale. It is also known as expanding symmetry or evolving symmetry. If the replication is exactly the same at every scale, it is called a self-similar pattern. An example of

this is the Menger Sponge. Fractals can also be nearly the same at different levels. Fractals also include the idea of a detailed pattern that repeats itself. The term "fractal" was first used by mathematician Benoit Mandelbrot in 1975.

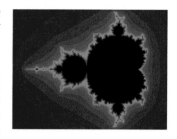

Fractals are different from other geometric figures because of the way in which they scale. Doubling the edge lengths of a polygon multiplies its area by four, which is two (the ratio of the new to the old side length) raised to the power of two (the dimension of the space the polygon resides in). Likewise, if the radius of a sphere is doubled, its volume scales by eight, which is two (the ratio of the new to the old radius) to the power of three (the dimension that the sphere resides in). (clearlyexplained.com)

Franklin, Rosalind Elsie (July 25, 1920 – April 16, 1958)
Franklin was an English chemist and X-ray crystallographer who made contributions to the understanding of the molecular structures of DNA (deoxyribonucleic acid), RNA (ribonucleic acid), viruses, coal, and graphite. Although her works on coal and viruses were appreciated in her lifetime, her contributions to the discovery of the structure of DNA were largely recognized posthumously.

Born to a prominent British Jewish family, Franklin was educated at private schools in London. She studied the Natural Sciences Tripos at Newnham College, Cambridge, from which she graduated in 1941. Earning a research fellowship, she joined the University of Cambridge physical chemistry laboratory. The British Coal Utilization Research Association (BCURA) offered her a research position in 1942, and started her work on coals. She earned a Ph.D. in 1945. She went to Paris in 1947 as a chercheur (post-doctoral researcher) under Jacques Mering at the Laboratoire Central des Services Chimiques de l'Etat, where she became an accomplished X-ray crystallographer. She became a research associate at King's College London in 1951 and worked on X-ray diffraction studies, which would eventually facilitate the double helix theory of the DNA. She died in 1958 at the age of 37 of ovarian cancer.

Franklin is best known for her work on the X-ray diffraction images of DNA, particularly Photo 51, while at King's College, London, which led to the discovery of the DNA double helix for which James Watson, Francis Crick and Maurice Wilkins shared the Nobel Prize in Physiology or Medicine in 1962. Watson suggested that Franklin would have ideally been awarded a Nobel Prize in Chemistry, along with Wilkins, but the Nobel Committee does not make posthumous nominations.

After finishing her work on DNA, Franklin led pioneering work at Birkbeck on the molecular structures of viruses. Her team member Aaron Klug continued her research, winning the Nobel Prize in Chemistry in 1982. (www.biography.com)

Gauge bosons
In particle physics, a gauge boson is a force carrier, a bosonic particle that carries any of the fundamental interactions of nature, commonly called forces. Elementary particles, whose interactions are described by a gauge theory, interact with each other by the exchange of gauge bosons—usually as virtual particles. All known gauge bosons have a spin of 1. Therefore, all known gauge bosons are vector bosons. Gauge bosons are different from the other kinds of bosons: first, fundamental scalar bosons (the Higgs boson); second, mesons, which are composite bosons, made of quarks; third, larger composite, non-force-carrying bosons, such as certain atoms. (The Info List – Gauge Boson)

Golden Ratio
The Golden ratio is a special number found by dividing a line into two parts so that the longer part divided by the smaller part is also equal to the whole length divided by the longer part. It is often symbolized using phi, after the 21st letter of the Greek alphabet.

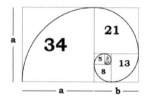

Some twentieth-century artists and architects, including Da Vinci, Le Corbusier and Dali, have proportioned their works to approximate the golden ratio—especially in the form of the golden rectangle, in which the ratio of the longer side to the shorter is the golden ratio—believing this proportion to be aesthetically pleasing. The golden ratio appears in some patterns in nature, including the spiral arrangement of leaves and other plant parts. (www.lifescience.com)

Mathematicians since Euclid have studied the properties of the golden ratio, including its appearance in the dimensions of a regular pentagon and in a golden rectangle, which may be cut into a square and a smaller rectangle with the same aspect ratio.

Grassroots Health
A Consortium of Scientists, Institutions and Individuals Committed to Solving the Worldwide Vitamin D Deficiency Epidemic.

Gurwitsch, Alexander (1874 – 1954)

Gurwitsch was a Russian and Soviet biologist and medical scientist who originated the morphogenetic field theory and discovered the biophoton. Gurwitsch was Professor of Histology and Embryology at Moscow University from 1924 to 1929.

He then directed a laboratory at the Institute of Experimental Medicine in Leningrad from 1930 until 1945. He sought to redefine his "heretical" concept of the morphogenetic field in general essays, pointing to molecular interactions unexplained by chemistry. In 1941 he was awarded a Stalin Prize for his mitogenetic radiation work since it had apparently led to a cheap and simple way of diagnosing cancer. He was awarded the Stalin Prize in 1941 for his mitogenic radiation work. (wikivisually.com)

Holick, Michael F. (1946-)

Holick is an American endocrinologist, specializing in the field of vitamin D, such as the identification of both calcidiol, the major circulating form of vitamin D, and calcitriol, the active form of vitamin D. His work has been the basis for diagnostic tests and therapies for vitamin D-related diseases. He is a professor of medicine at the Boston University Medical Center and editor-in-chief of the journal Clinical Laboratory. (drholick.com)

Human Genome

The human genome is stored on 23 chromosome pairs in the cell nucleus and in the small mitochondrial DNA. A great deal is now known about the sequences of DNA which are on our chromosomes. What the DNA actually does is now partly known. Applying this knowledge in practice has only just begun.

The Human Genome Project (HGP) produced a reference sequence which is used worldwide in biology and medicine. The latest project ENCODE studies the way the genes are controlled. (www.newworldencyclopedia.org)

The human genome contains just over 20,000 protein-coding genes, far fewer than had been expected. In fact, only about 1.5 percent of the genome codes for proteins, while the rest consists of non-coding RNA genes, regulatory sequences, and introns.

With RNA splicing and post-RNA translation changes, the total number of unique human proteins may be in the low millions.

Huldschinsky, Kurt (1883 – December 15, 1940)

Huldschinsky was a German Pediatrician of Polish heritage (Prussian). He served in the Wehrmacht as a field medic in World War I. Later, as a medical doctor and research scientist, he successfully demonstrated in the winter of 1918/1919 how rickets could be treated with ultraviolet lamps. At that time perhaps half of all German children suffered from rickets. It was already understood that this disease was caused by a calcium deficiency. Up to that point, heliotherapy was a common protocol for many illnesses and showed promise in relieving the effects of rickets. The biochemical mechanism triggered in the human dermis by the sun's electromagnetic radiation was not fully understood, and scientists were exploring mostly the long wavelength (red) end of the spectrum. To generate artificial UV, Dr. Huldschinsky originally tried to adapt existing X-Ray technology.(Wikipedia)

Integumentary system

The integumentary system is the organ system that protects the body from various kinds of damage, such as loss of water or abrasion from outside. The system comprises the skin and its appendages (including hair, scales, feathers, hooves, and nails).

The integumentary system has a variety of functions; it may serve to waterproof, cushion, and protect the deeper tissues, excrete wastes, and regulate temperature, and is the attachment site for sensory receptors to detect pain, sensation, pressure, and temperature. In most terrestrial vertebrates with significant exposure to sunlight, the integumentary system also provides for vitamin D synthesis. (Wikipedia)

Leprosy

Leprosy is a long-term infection by the bacteria Mycobacterium leprae or Mycobacterium lepromatosis. Initially, infections are without symptoms and typically remain this way for 5 to 20 years. Symptoms that develop include granulomas of the nerves, respiratory tract, skin, and eyes. This may result in a lack of ability to feel pain, thus loss of parts of extremities due to repeated injuries or infection due to unnoticed wounds. Weakness and poor eyesight may also be present. Leprosy is spread between people. Leprosy occurs more commonly among those living in poverty. Contrary to popular belief, it is not highly contagious. (Wikipedia)

Microtubule (micro + tube + ule)

Microtubules are a component of the cytoskeleton, found throughout the cytoplasm. These tubular polymers of tubulin can grow as long as 50 micrometers and are highly dynamic. The outer diameter of a microtubule is about 24 nm while the inner diameter is about

12 nm. They are found in eukaryotic cells, as well as some bacteria, and are formed by the polymerization of a dimer of two globular proteins, alpha and beta tubulin.

Microtubules are very important in a number of cellular processes. They are involved in maintaining the structure of the cell and, together with microfilaments and intermediate filaments, they form the cytoskeleton. They also make up the internal structure of cilia and flagella. They provide platforms for intracellular transport and are involved in a variety of cellular processes, including the movement of secretory vesicles, organelles, and intracellular macromolecular assemblies. They are also involved in chromosome separation (mitosis and meiosis), and are the major constituents of mitotic spindles, which are used to pull apart eukaryotic chromosomes.

Microtubules are nucleated and organized by microtubule organizing centers (MTOCs), such as the centrosome found in the center of many animal cells or the basal bodies found in cilia and flagella, or the spindle pole bodies found in most fungi.

There are many proteins that bind to microtubules, including the motor proteins kinesin and dynein, severing proteins like katanin, and other proteins important for regulating microtubule dynamics. (*Foundation in Microbiology*)

Mitosis
Mitosis is the usual method of cell division, characterized typically by the resolving of the chromatin of the nucleus into a threadlike form, which condenses into chromosomes, each of which separates longitudinally into two parts, one part of each chromosome being retained in each of two new cells resulting from the original cell. Mitosis is the type of cell division in which one cell divides into two cells that are exactly the same, each with the same number of chromosomes as the original cell.

Pollack, Dr. Gerald
Pollack is a professor of bioengineering at the University of Washington, the founder and editor-in-chief of a scientific journal called Water, and author of many peer-reviewed scientific papers on the topic of water. He has received prestigious awards from the National Institutes of Health.

The fourth phase of water is, in a nutshell, living water. It's referred to as EZ water—EZ standing for "exclusion zone"—which has a negative charge. This water can hold energy, much like a battery, and can deliver energy too.

The key to Dr. Pollack's entire hypothesis lies in the properties of water. The water molecules become structured in arrays or strata when they interact with charged surfaces such as those presented by proteins. The cell's water is potentially structured. Water stays put in the cells because it's absorbed into the protein surfaces. Structured water adheres to the proteins of the cells.

Structured water does not have the same properties as bulk water. Water is the carrier of the most important molecules of life, like proteins and DNA. In the book, *Cells, Gels and the Engines of Life*, evidence is presented that shows water is absolutely essential to everything the cell does. The water in our cells is actually ordered pretty much like a crystal. Like ice, it excludes particles and solutes as it forms. Pollack sees EZ water as healing water. (mercola.com)

Books: *The Fourth Phase of Water*: Beyond Solid, Liquid, and Vapor and *Cells, Gels and the Engines of Life*.

Popp, Dr. Fritz Albert (1938 – 2010)
Popp is a German philosopher and researcher in biophysics, particularly in the study of biophotons. His first diploma was in Experimental Physics (1966, University Würzburg), followed by the Roentgen Prize of the University Würzburg, Ph.D. in Theoretical Physics (1969, University Mainz). Habilitation in Biophysics and Medicine (1973, University Marburg). Prof. Popp rediscovered and made the first extensive physical analysis of "Biophotons." He lectured at Marburg University from 1973 to 1980. He was head of a research group in the Pharmaceutical Industry in Worms from 1981 to 1983 and head of a research group at the Institute of Cell Biology (University Kaiserslautern) from 1983 to 1986 and of another research group at the Technology Center in Kaiserslautern.

Popp has conducted research confirming the existence of biophotons. These particles of light, with no mass, transmit information within and between cells. His work shows that DNA in living cell stores and releases photons creating "biophotonic emissions" that may hold the key to illness and health. Popp's eight books and more than 150 scientific journal articles and studies address basic questions of theoretical physics, biology, complementary medicine and biophotons. (Int. Institute of Biophysics)

Redox potential
Reduction potential is a measure of the tendency of a chemical species to acquire electrons and thereby be reduced. Reduction potential is measured in volts (V), or millivolts (mV). Each species has its own intrinsic reduction potential; the more positive the potential, the greater the species' affinity for electrons and tendency to be reduced. Oxidation Reduction Potential (ORP) is a common measurement for water quality. (www.biology-pages.info)

Resonance

In physics, resonance is a phenomenon in which a vibrating system or external force drives another system to oscillate with greater amplitude at a specific preferential frequency. The term resonance (from Latin resonantia, 'echo', from resonare, 'resound') originates from the field of acoustics, particularly observed in musical instruments, e.g., when strings started to vibrate and to produce sound without direct excitation by the player. (Wikipedia)

Resonance occurs when a system is able to store and easily transfer energy between two or more different storage modes (such as kinetic energy and potential energy in the case of a pendulum). Resonance phenomena occur with all types of vibrations or waves: there is mechanical resonance, acoustic resonance, electromagnetic resonance, nuclear magnetic resonance (NMR), electron spin resonance (ESR), and resonance of quantum wave functions. Resonant systems can be used to generate vibrations of a specific frequency (e.g., musical instruments), or pick out specific frequencies from a complex vibration containing many frequencies (e.g., filters).

Resonance occurs widely in nature, and is exploited in many manmade devices. It is the mechanism by which virtually all sinusoidal waves and vibrations are generated. Many sounds we hear, such as when hard objects of metal, glass, or wood are struck, are caused by brief resonant vibrations in the object. Light and other short wavelength electromagnetic radiation is produced by resonance on an atomic scale, such as electrons in atoms. (www.concepts.org)

RNA

Ribonucleic acid (RNA) is a linear molecule composed of four types of smaller molecules called ribonucleotide bases: adenine (A), cytosine (C), guanine (G), and uracil (U). RNA is often compared to a copy from a reference book, or a template, because it carries the same information as its DNA template but is not used for long-term storage. RNA is synthesized from DNA by an enzyme known as RNA polymerase during a process called transcription. The new RNA sequences are complementary to their DNA template, rather than being identical copies of the template. RNA is then translated into proteins by structures called ribosomes. There are three types of RNA involved in the translation process: messenger RNA (mRNA), transfer RNA (tRNA), and ribosomal RNA (rRNA). Although some RNA molecules are passive copies of DNA, many play crucial, active roles in the cell. For example, some RNA molecules are involved in switching genes on and off, and other RNA molecules make up the critical protein synthesis machinery in ribosomes. (www.nature.com)

Schauberger, Victor (1885 - 1958)

Schauberger was an Austrian forest caretaker, naturalist, philosopher, and inventor. Schauberger developed his own ideas based on what he observed in nature. One of his inventions is the "trout turbine." His understanding was built up from shamanic and experiential observation of Nature in the untamed Alpine wilderness. His motto: "Observe and Copy Nature." Schauberger was also gifted with engineering skills which are apparent in his environment-friendly technology and implosive energy devices designed to release people from enslavement to destructive sources of energy. He is known for his discoveries in the water sciences, in agricultural techniques and in the energy domain.

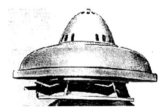

During World War II, Victor Schauberger was interned in a Nazi concentration camp and was forced to work on a flying disk project using his ideas. After World War II, Viktor emigrated to the United States on promises by various agencies (CIA) to help him develop and test his ideas. He went to a facility in Dallas Texas, and under uncertain direction, signed over all of the rights to his inventions and patents to the US government. He was sent back to his homeland of Austria only to die, broken and disillusioned, five days later.

An original picture-sketch of the Repulsine above right: A flying model of a Schauberger Repulsine, Type A, tested in January 1940. This device has been built with copper and uses a very high speed motor for the main vortex turbine. (www.vortex-world.org)

Schrödinger, Erwin Rudolf Josef Alexander (August 12, 1887 –January 4, 1961)

Schrödinger was a Nobel Prize-winning Austrian physicist who developed a number of fundamental results in the field of quantum theory, which formed the basis of wave mechanics. He formulated the wave equation (stationary and time-dependent Schrödinger equation) and revealed the identity of his development of the formalism and matrix mechanics. Schrödinger proposed an original interpretation of the physical meaning of the wave function. (Wikipedia)

In addition, he was the author of many works in various fields of physics: statistical mechanics and thermodynamics, physics of dielectrics, color theory, electrodynamics, general relativity, and cosmology, and he made several attempts to construct a unified field theory. In his book *What Is Life?* Schrödinger addressed the problems of genetics, looking at the phenomenon of life from the point of view of physics. He paid great attention to the philosophical aspects of science, ancient and oriental philosophical concepts, ethics, and religion. He also wrote on philosophy and theoretical biology. He is also known for his "Schrödinger's cat" thought-experiment.

Soliton light wave

The storage of light and information in the DNA takes place is in the form of a special light wave, called Soliton wave. This wave encases the DNA molecule. It is a nonlinear waveform, which follows very complicated laws, the so-called Fermi-Pasta-Ulam grid. Soliton waves are extremely durable and hardly change shape. They are therefore suited to store information patterns over a long period and also to transport over long distances. In August 1834, John Scott Russell discovered the soliton wave. He was riding beside the Union Canal near Edinburgh, Scotland; he noticed a strange wave building up at the bow of a boat. After the boat stopped, the wave travelled on, "assuming the form of a large solitary elevation, a rounded, smooth and well-defined heap of water, which continued its course along the channel apparently without change of form or diminution of speed." (Department of Mathematics www.macs.hw.ac.uk)

Schumann, Otto

German physicist Winfried Otto Schumann documented the Schumann Resonance in 1952. He understood that global electromagnetic resonances exist within the cavity between the Earth's surface and the inner edge of the ionosphere and are excited and activated by lightning. Schumann resonances were first measured reliably in the early 1960s. Schumann's then doctoral student Herbert König made extensive measurements and was able to establish the exact value of this earth resonance frequency at 7.83 hertz. This value has since been generally referred to as Schumann frequency in science. Since then, scientists have discovered that variations in the resonances correspond to changes in the seasons, solar activity, activity in Earth's magnetic environment, in water aerosols in the atmosphere, and other Earth-bound phenomena. (Wikipedia)

Sumer and Sumerian Civilization

Sumer was the southernmost region of ancient Mesopotamia (modern-day Iraq and Kuwait) which is generally considered the cradle of civilization. The name comes from Akkadian, the language of the north of Mesopotamia, and means "land of the civilized kings." The Sumerians called themselves "the black headed people" and their land, in cuneiform script, was simply "the land" or "the land of the black headed people." According to the Sumerian King List, when the gods first gave human beings the gifts necessary for cultivating society, they did so by establishing the city of Eridu in the region of Sumer. While the Sumerian city of Uruk is held to be the oldest city in the world, the ancient Mesopotamians believed that it was Eridu and that it was here that order was established and civilization began. Sumer was the birthplace of writing, the wheel, agriculture, the arch, the plow, irrigation, and many other innovations. The 360 degree circle, the foot and its 12 inches, and the "dozen" as a unit, are but a few examples of the vestiges of Sumerian mathematics, still evident in our daily lives.

The Sumerians are amongst the first people to leave sophisticated records of their astronomical observations. Their fascination with the heavens is apparent in the large number of seals and cuneiform tablets unearthed of an astronomical nature. The Sumerians were the first to divide both space and time by units of six. The modern division of the year into 12 months, the 24 hours of each day, the division of hours into 60 minutes and 60 seconds, and the divisions of the circle/sphere by 360 degrees, each composed of 60 minutes and 60 seconds of an arc, are all Sumerian developments. (www.ancient.eu)

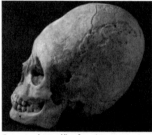

Chemical analysis has identified a 6,000-year-old brewery at an archaeological site in what is now modern Iran. The evidence suggests that fermentation of barley was first practiced in Sumer - southern Babylonia - between 4000 and 3000 BC.

The earliest significant record of skull elongation comes in the form of the pottery representations of the Gods from the 5th millennium B.C. The Al-Ubaid culture proceeded the Sumerian culture was a people known as the Ubaidians who established settlements in the region later known as Sumer (Mesopotamia).

Source: http://beforeitsnews.com

Szent-Gyorgyi, Albert Imre (1893 - 1986)

The Hungarian-born biochemist was the first to isolate vitamin C. His research on biological oxidation provided the basis for Krebs' citric acid cycle. His discoveries about the biochemical nature of muscular contraction revolutionized the field of muscle research. His later career was devoted to research in "sub-molecular" biology, applying quantum physics to biological processes. He was especially interested in cancer, and was one of the first to explore the connections between free radicals and cancer. Szent-Gyorgyi won the 1937 Nobel Prize in Physiology or Medicine for his work in biological oxidation and vitamin C, and the Lasker Award in Basic Medical Research in 1954, for contributions to understanding cardiovascular disease through basic muscle research. (www.encyclopedia.com)

Tablet of Shamash
This is a stone tablet recovered from the ancient Babylonian city of Sippar in southern Iraq in 1881; it is now a major piece in the British Museum's ancient Middle East collection. It is dated to the reign of King Nabu-apla-iddina ca. 888 – 855 BC.

Tesla, Nikola (July 10, 1856 –January 7, 1943)
Tesla was a Serbian-American inventor, electrical engineer, mechanical engineer, physicist, and futurist who is best known for his contributions to the design of the modern alternating current (AC) electricity supply system. Born and raised in the Austrian Empire, Tesla received an advanced education in engineering and physics in the 1870s and gained practical experience in the early 1880s working in telephony and at Continental Edison in the new electric power industry. Emigrating to the United States in 1884, where he would become naturalized citizen, Tesla worked for a short time at Edison in New York City before he struck out on his own. With the help of partners to finance and market his ideas, Tesla set up laboratories and companies in New York to develop a range of electrical and mechanical devices. His alternating current (AC) induction motor and related polyphase AC patents, licensed by Westinghouse Electric in 1888, earned him a considerable amount of money and became the cornerstone of the polyphase system that company would eventually market.

Attempting to develop inventions he could patent and market, Tesla conducted a range of experiments with mechanical oscillators/generators, electrical discharge tubes, and early X-ray imaging. He also built a wireless-controlled boat, one of the first ever exhibited. (www.encyclopedia.com)

Throughout the 1890s Tesla would pursue his ideas for wireless lighting and worldwide wireless electric power distribution in his high-voltage, high-frequency power experiments in New York and Colorado Springs. Early on (1893) he made pronouncements on the possibility of wireless communication with his devices. He tried to put these ideas to practical use in his unfinished Wardenclyffe Tower project, an intercontinental wireless communication and power transmitter, but ran out of funding before he could complete it. (Nikola Tesla Society)

Inventions:
- Alternating Current – The DC current that Edison (backed by General Electric) had been working on was costly over long distances, and produced dangerous sparking from the required converter. Alternating Current is perfectly safe. Tesla's system that provides power generation and distribution to North America in our modern era.
- Light – Tesla did invent how light can be harnessed and distributed. Tesla developed and used fluorescent bulbs in his lab some 40 years before industry "invented" them.
- X-rays – Tesla played a central role in developing X-ray systems.
- Radio – it is proven that Tesla invented the radio years previous to Marconi.
- Remote Control – Tesla considered this invention a natural outcropping of radio.
- Electric Motor –Tesla's invented a motor with rotating magnetic fields. The first car to run on this type of motor was the 1934 Pierce Arrow.
- Robotics – Nikola Tesla's overly enhanced scientific mind led him to the idea that all living beings are merely driven by external impulses. This was the begin of robotics research.
- Laser –Lasers have transformed surgical applications in an undeniably beneficial way, and they have given rise to much of our current digital media.
- Wireless communications and limitless free energy – Tesla represented the world's first wireless communications. Tesla was dedicated to empowering the individual to receive and transmit this data virtually free of charge.

Wave-particle duality
In physics and chemistry, wave-particle duality holds that light and matter exhibit properties of both waves and of particles. A central concept of quantum mechanics, wave-particle duality addresses the inadequacy of conventional concepts like "particle" and "wave" to meaningfully describe the behavior of quantum objects. The idea of duality is rooted in a debate over the nature of light and matter dating back to the 1600s, when competing theories of light were proposed by Christiaan Huygens and Isaac Newton. Through the work of Albert Einstein, Louis de Broglie and many others, it is now established that all objects have both wave and particle nature, and that a suitable interpretation of quantum mechanics provides the over-arching theory resolving this ostensible paradox. (www.science.daily.com)

Wormhole
A wormhole is a "tube made of space time" that connects two different regions. If it is set up right, you could enter one side of the tube and exit the other end somewhere else, or even some when else. In contrast, a black hole destroys all things, and doesn't "go anywhere."

A wormhole is a funnel (what's shown here is only a two dimensional funnel) that tapers down to a "throat" (which although thinner never pinches off entirely) which connects to another funnel that opens up somewhere else. A black hole is a funnel that pinches off at a singularity. A traversable wormhole needs to be large and "mellow" enough that it doesn't have an event horizon (a black hole's "point of no return"), or any fatal tidal forces.

Einstein's work was at the heart of the theory of wormholes, or "bridges" as he called them. The idea of a hypothetical topological feature of spacetime that is essentially a shortcut through space and time, potentially linking widely separated parts of the universe (or even different universes), has been understandably much loved by science fiction writers over the years, although there is also much theoretical work to support them. (www.quora.com)

Sources of photo material:

archive
123 rf stockfoto
Fotolia
dreamstime
other references are given

Author: Irmgard Maria Gräf

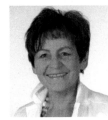

Born in Germany, Irmgard M. Gräf spent many years with her husband and five children in Huntsville, Alabama, heart of ancient Indian cultures and also the center of the manned space program. From American Indians she learned their philosophy and immense respect for all life forms. She studied alternate medicine and many connected therapies. Due to her husband's work at NASA she challenged her analytical mind in great conversations with genius minds, scientists and astronauts. She grew accustomed to seeking out the newest and perhaps controversial developments in the field of science. She directed a privately owned Nikola Tesla school and taught there.

Back in Europe, Irmgard Gräf decided to expand her nutritional and therapeutic background and work professionally as a certified dietitian. Nutrition is the foundation of life to her. Her love and trust in nature's power is constantly balanced through investigative thinking. Medicine and quantum physics are her passion.

Books and publications:
- *Die Quark-Öl-Kur – Die Heilwirkungen der Öl-Eiweiss-Kost nach Dr. Budwig*, (The oil-protein cure - The healing effects of the oil protein diet according to Dr. Budwig) ViaNova Verlag 2014 (26)
- *Mein Blut ein Weg zu mir – was mein Blut mir sagt* (My blood – a key to personal health) Michaels Verlag 2014 (454)
- *Blut – Datenhighway* (Data highway of your blood) Matrix 3000, 2015, Bd. 86
- *Stoffwechsel – Brücke zwischen Körper und Seele* (Metabolism – bridge between body and soul) Matrix 3000

She writes articles in professional journals and lectures in academies in Germany, Switzerland, and Liechtenstein

Educational background:
University of Alabama in Huntsville, U.S.A; RSE, WA U.S.A.; Reformhaus Academy, Germany; Institute Vitamin Delta, Germany; Dr. Budwig Academy, Germany.

References:

1. **Lillge, Wolfgang M.D.** Biophysics And the Life Process. *21st Centura Science & Technology Magazine.* [Online] 2001. http://www.21stcenturysciencetech.com/articles/summ01/Biophysics/Biophysics.html.

2. **Gurwitsch, A.** *Das Problem der Zellteilung (the problem of cell division).* s.l. : Springer-Verlag, 1926. ISBN-13: 978-3642888052.

3. **Schrödinger, Erwin.** *What is Life - With Mind and Matter and Autobiographical Sketches (Canto Classics).* s.l. : Cambridge University Press Auflage: Reprint , 2012 Reprint.

4. **Eden, Dan.** Is DNA the next internet? *mondovista.* [Online] http://mondovista.com/dnax.html.

5. Biophotonics – The Science Behind Energy Healing. *The Event Chronicle.* [Online] Sep 21, 2015. http://www.theeventchronicle.com/metaphysics/metascience/biophotonics-the-science-behind-energy-healing/.

6. **Schwabl,Herbert , Herbert Klima.** living-systems-give-measurable-intensities-light-ie-photons-visible-part-electromagnetic. *Green Med Info.* [Online] Forsch Komplementarmed Klass Naturheilkd. 2005 Apr;12(2):84-9. PMID: 15947466, 2005. http://www.greenmedinfo.com/article/living-systems-give-measurable-intensities-light-ie-photons-visible-part-electromagnetic.

7. **Popp, Prof. Dr. Fritz Albert.** We know today that man, essentially, is a being of light.". *Biophotonservice.* [Online] 2012. http://biophotonservices.com/dr-fritz-albert-popp/.

8. **Gribbin, John.** *Q is for Quantum - An Encyclopedia of Particle Physics.* New York : s.n., 1998.

9. **Camejo, Silvia Arroyo.** *Skurile Quantenwelten.* Heidelberg : s.n., 2006.

10. We are beings of light. [Online] May 15, 2016. http://i9bottle.com/the-human-body-emits-and-communicates-with-biophotons-we-are-beings-of-light-as-well/.

11. **Watkins, Alan.** *Coherence: The secret Science of Brilliant leadership.* 1961. ISBN: 978-0-7494-7005-0.

12. We are beings of light. *i9bottle.com.* [Online] May 15, 2016. http://i9bottle.com/the-human-body-emits-and-communicates-with-biophotons-we-are-beings-of-light-as-well/.

13. **Popp, Prof. Dr. Fritz Albert.** Der Mensch ist ein Lichtsäuger. *Naturscheck.* [Online] 2010. http://www.naturscheck.de/artikel/artikel-interviews/interviews/prof_dr_fritz_a_popp__der_mensch_ist_ein_lichtsaeuger.

14. **Garajev Dr. Peter, Poponin Vladimir.** Dr. Peter Garajev & Vladimir Poponin - DNA BioComputer Reprogramming. *rex serearch.* [Online] http://www.rexresearch.com/gajarev/gajarev.htm.

15. **Sun Y, Wang C, Dai J.** Biophotons as neural communication signals demonstrated by in situ biophoton autography. *PubMed.* [Online] March 2010. https://www.ncbi.nlm.nih.gov/pubmed/20221457.

16. **Morgan, Edward.** Scientific Experiments Show That DNA Begins as a Quantum Wave and Not as a Molecule. *Prepare for change.* [Online] Feb 4, 2017. http://prepareforchange.net/2017/02/04/scientific-experiments-show-that-dna-begins-as-a-quantum-wave-and-not-as-a-molecule/.

17. **Pumtiwitt, C., McCarthy.** Everything is illuminated: 'Reflections' on light and life by Lubert Stryer. [Online] Oct 2012. http://www.asbmb.org/asbmbtoday/asbmbtoday_article.aspx?id=18029.

18. **Wilz, Gregor, Wunsch Alexander.** *Licht Therapie, die medizin der Zukunft.* s.l. : ViaNova Verlag, 2017. ISBN: 978-3-86616-371-3.

19. **Ming.** World Transformation: Biophotons And The Universal Light Code. [Online] May 1, 2004. http://www.worldtrans.org/newslog2.html/__show_article/_a000002-000110.htm.

20. **Popp, Dr. Fritz Albert.** *Biophotons Popp Interview Part 1.* 2011.

21. **Alberts, Bruce, Alexander Johnson, Julian Lewis, Martin Raff, Keith Roberts, and Peter Walter.** *Molecular Biology of the Cell, 4th edition.* s.l. : Garland Science, 2002. ISBN-10: 0-8153-4072-9.

22. **Budwig, Dr. Johanna.** Das Fettsyndrom. *Dr. Johanna Budwig und die Öl-Eiweiss-Kost.* [Online] http://www.oel-eiweiss-kost.de/_oel_eiweiss_kost/_oekost_hinweise.html.

23. **Donner, Dipl. rer nat Susanne.** Biophotonen: Mehr Licht - mehr Qualität. *UGB.* [Online] 2014. https://www.ugb.de/forschung-studien/biophotonen-mehr-licht-mehr-qualitaet/.

24. **Galle, Michael.** Die MORA Resonanztherapie. *Diagcenter.* [Online] Jan 2007. http://www.diagcenter.si/dokumenti/studije/mora-medicine/MORA-Galle2007-Ubersicht-MORA-Therapie.pdf.

25. **Grashorn MA, Ulrike Egerer.** Integrated assessment of quality organic eggs by measurement of dark luminescence. [Online] polish journal of food and nutrition sciences, 2007. agro.icm.edu.pl/agro/element/...element.agro.../praca_035_191-1.

26. **Gräf, Irmgard Maria.** *Die Quark-Öl-Kur. Die Heilkraft der Öl-Eiweiss-Ernährung nach Dr. Budwig.* s.l. : ViaNova Verlag, 2014.

27. **Kuzemsky, A.L.** BIOGRAPHY OF Herbert Frohlich (1905 - 1991). *thero.jinr.* [Online] 2012. http://theor.jinr.ru/~kuzemsky/hfrobio.html.

28. Ilya Prigogine - Biographical. *The Nobel Prize in Chemistry 1977.* [Online] 1977. http://www.nobelprize.org/nobel_prizes/chemistry/laureates/1977/prigogine-bio.html.

29. The History of DNA Timeline. *DNA Worldwide.* [Online] Aug 2003. https://www.dna-worldwide.com/resource/160/history-dna-timeline.

30. **Pray, Leslie A. Ph.D.** Discovery of DNA Structure and Function: Watson and Crick. *Nature Education.* [Online] 2008. http://www.nature.com/scitable/topicpage/discovery-of-dna-structure-and-function-watson-discovery-of-dna-structure-and-function-watson-discovery-of-dna-structure-and-function-watson-discovery-of-dna-structure-and-function-watson-discovery-of-dna-structure.

31. The discovery of DNA. *your genome.org.* [Online] http://www.yourgenome.org/stories/the-discovery-of-dna.

32. Erwin Chargaff. *famous scientists.* [Online] https://www.famousscientists.org/erwin-chargaff/.

33. **Chargaff, Erwin.** *Heraclitean Fire.* s.l. : Springer, 1975. ISBN-13: 978-0874700299.

34. James Watson, Francis Crick, Maurice Wilkins, and Rosalind Franklin. *Chemical Heritage Foundation.* [Online] https://www.chemheritage.org/historical-profile/james-watson-francis-crick-maurice-wilkins-and-rosalind-franklin.

35. **Mandal, Ananya M.D., Cashin-Garbutt.** History of DNA Research. [Online] 2006. http://www.news-medical.net/life-sciences/History-of-DNA-Research.aspx.

36. **Wilcock, David.** *The synchronicity Key: the Hidden Intelligence Guiding the Universse and You.* s.l. : Dutton; Reprint edition (July 29, 2014), 2014. ISBN-13: 978-0142181089.

37. **Shuttler, Lance.** New Science: DNA Begins As a Quantum Wave. *The Mind Unleashed.* [Online] 2017. http://themindunleashed.com/2017/01/new-science-dna-begins-quantum-wave.html.

38. —. Scientific Experiments Show That DNA Begins as a Quantum Wave and Not as a Molecule. *Omnithought.org.* [Online] Feb 2, 2017. http://omnithought.org/scientific-experiments-show-dna-begins-as-quantum-wave-not-as-molecule/5279.

39. **Fosar, G., F. Bludorf.** *Vernetzte Intelligenz.* s.l. : Omega, 2006. ISBN-13: 978-3930243235.

40. The Human Genome Project Completion. *NIH National Human Genome Research Institute.* [Online] 2003. https://www.genome.gov/11006943/human-genome-project-completion-frequently-asked-questions/.

41. **Popp, F.A. Prof. Dr.** *Coherent photon storage of biological systems .* Wien-Baltimore : Electro-magnetic Bioinformation, 1979.

42. **Bludorf, Fosar Grazyna and Franz.** Rex Research. *http://rexresearch.com/gajarev/gajarev.htm.* [Online]

43. **Pitkänen, Matti.** *Wormholes and possible new physics in biological length scales.* Helsinki : s.n., 1997.

44. ZEIT online. *http://www.zeit.de/wissen/geschichte/2011-07/physiker-wheeler.* [Online] 2011.

45. **Kaku, Michio.** *Hyperspace: A Scientific Odyssey through Parallel Universes, Time Warps, and the Tenth Dimension .* Oxford : s.n., 1995.

46. **Staughton, John.** What are wormholes? *Science ABC.* [Online] https://www.scienceabc.com/nature/universe/what-are-wormholes-einstein-rosen-bridge-theory-possible-real.html.

47. Russian DNA Research. [Online] http://www.nrgnair.com/MPT/zdi_tech/DNA.research.htm.

48. In the human brain discovered quantum tunnel. *The Newspapers Gthering and spreading news from various Russin newspapers.* [Online] Jul 20, 2016. http://the-newspapers.com/2016/07/20/in-the-human-brain-discovered-quantum-tunnel.

49. **Collins, Andrew.** *Cygnus Mystery: Unlocking the Ancient Secret of Life's Origins in the Cosmos.* s.l. : Watkins Publishing, 1999. ISBN-13: 978-1906787554.

50. **Kingsley.** Between both worlds. *http://betweenbothworlds.blogspot.ch/2010/10/quantum-consciousness-3-hyper.html.* [Online] 2010.

51. **Anthony, Peake.** *Infinite Mindfield: A Quest to Find the Gateway to Higher Consciousness.* London : Watkins Publishing , 2013. ISBN-13: 978-1780285719.

52. **Bradon, Gregg.** *The phantom experience Vladimir Poponin.* [youtube] https://www.youtube.com/watch?v=PUdgAknS700 : s.n., 2011.

53. Famous Dreams. *www.dreaminetrpretation-dictionnary.com.* [Online] http://www.dreaminterpretation-dictionary.com/famous-dreams-paul-mccartney.html.

54. **Bludorf, Fosar Graznya and Franz.** Crawford. *http://www.bibliotecapleyades.net/ciencia/ciencia_genetica02.htm.* [Online] 2002.

55. **Sheldrake, Rupert.** *Dogs That Know When Their Owners Are Coming Home: Fully Updated and Revised.* s.l. : Broadway Books, 2011. Dogs That Know When Their Owners Are Coming Home: Fully Updated and Revised.

56. **Garajev, Peter Ph.D.** Wave Genetics. *WAve Genetics.* [Online] http://eng.wavegenetic.ru/index.php?option=com_content&task=view&id=2&itemid=1.

57. Groundbreaking Russian DNA Discoveries. *DIVINE COSMOS.* [Online] Oct 10, 2007. http://divinecosmos.com/start-here/articles/362-groundbreaking-russian-dna-discoveries.

58. **Soljacic, Marin , Suzanne Sears, Mordechai Segev,Dmitriy Krylov, and Keren Bergman.** Self-Similarity and Fractals Driven by Soliton Dynamics. *mit.edu.* [Online] http://www.mit.edu/~soljacic/frac_euro_fin.pdf.

59. **Cosmos, Divine.** Groundbreaking Russian DNA Discoveries. *http://divinecosmos.com/start-here/articles/362-groundbreaking-russian-dna-discoveries.* [Online] 10 17, 2007.

60. **Blank M, Goodman R.** DNA is a fractal antenna in electromagnetic fields. *PubMed.* [Online] Apr 2011. https://www.ncbi.nlm.nih.gov/pubmed/21457072.

61. **P.P.Gariaev, G.G.Tertishny, A.M. Iarochenko, V.V.Maximenko, E.A.Leonova.** The spectroscopy of biophotons in non-local genetic regulation. *http://www.emergentmind.org/gariaevi3.htm.* [Online] 2001.

62. **Nature.** Nature chemistry. *http://www.nature.com/nchem/journal/v5/n3/full/nchem.1548.html.* [Online] 2012.

63. **Popopnin, Vladimir Dr.** The DNA Phantom Effect. *http://www.bibliotecapleyades.net/ciencia/ciencia_genetica04.htm.* [Online] 2001.

64. **Rein, Glen.** Frog embryo changed into a salamander. *http://www.keelynet.com/news/041914f.html.* [Online] 4 19, 2014.

65. **Coghlan, Andy.** Quadruple helix DNA discovered in human cells. *New Scientist.* [Online] Jan 23, 2013. https://www.newscientist.com/article/mg21729014-400-quadruple-helix-dna-discovered-in-human-cells/.

66. **Biffi, Giulia e.al.** Quantitative visuliszation of DNA G-quadruplexe structures in human cells. *http://www.nature.com/nchem/journal/v5/n3/full/nchem.1548.html*. [Online] 10 17, 2012.

67. Health Mail Online. *http://www.dailymail.co.uk/health/article-1375697/Alfie-Clamp-2-1st-person-born-extra-strand-DNA.html*. [Online] 3 11, 2011.

68. **Franckh, Pierre.** *The DNA Field and the Law of Resonance.* s.l. : Inner Tradition, 2014.

69. Gene expression. *http://iws.collin.edu/atassa/course-files/Biol_1408_Ch_11_3_Slide.pdf*. [Online] 2012.

70. Nature. *http://www.nature.com/scitable/topicpage/the-information-in-dna-is-decoded-by-6524808*. [Online] 2015.

71. **Lipton, Bruce H.Ph.D.** *Biology of belief.* s.l. : Hay House Inc. , 2011.

72. **Gräf, Irmgard Maria.** *Mein Blut – ein Weg zu mir .* Peiting : Michaels Verlag, 2014.

73. **Sniadeki.J.** *Sniadeki.J.See Mozolowski, W, 1939 Nature 1822; 143:121-12.* 1939.

74. **Zhang, Mingyong, Fan Shen,,Anna Petryk,Jingfeng Tang,Xingzhen Chen,and Consolato Serg.** "English Disease": Historical Notes on Rickets, the Bone–Lung Link and Child Neglect Issues. *Nutrients. ; 8(11): 722.* [Online] Nov 2016. https://www.ncbi.nlm.nih.gov/pmc/articles/PMC5133108/.

75. **Herbert Hönigsmann.** History of phototherapy in dermatology. *researchgate.* [Online] May 24, 2012. https://www.researchgate.net/publication/228081875_History_of_phototherapy_in_dermatology.

76. **Hess AF, Unger LL.** The cure of infantile rickets by sunlight. *Hess AF, Unger LL. The cure of infantile rickets by sunlight. JAMA 1921;77:39–41.* 1921.

77. Nature. *http://www.nature.com/bonekeyreports/2014/140108/bonekey2013212/full/bonekey2013212.html .* [Online] 2014.

78. **Campell, William Douglas II, MD.** *Into the Light, Tomorrows medicine Today.* Panama City : Rhino Publishing , 1993, 2003. ISBN 9962-636-27-2.

79. **Mc Collum, EV.** McCollum EV, Simmonds N, Becker JE, Shipley PG. An experimental demonstration of the existence of a vitamin which promotes calcium deposition. J Biol Chem 1922;53:293–298. *http://www.nature.com/bonekeyreports/2014/140108/bonekey2013213/full/bonekey2013213.html#ref21.* 1922.

80. **Nicolaysen, R.** The influence of vitamin D on the absorption of calcium and phosphorus in the rat. *Studies upon the mode of action of vitamin D. III. The influence of vitamin D on the absorption of calcium and phosphorus in the rat. Biochem J 1937;31:122–129.* 1937.

81. **Hulshinsky, K.** Heilung von rachitis durch künstlich hohen-sonne. . *Deut. Med. Wochenscher. 1919; 45: 712–713; Z. Orthopad. Chir. 1920; 39:426 as described in Bills CE. In: Sebrell WH Jr, Harris RS (eds). The Vitamins. Vol. II. Academic Press: New York, 1954,.* 1954.

82. openi.nlm.gov. *https://openi.nlm.nih.gov/detailedresult.php?img=PMC3897598_de-5-51-g88&req=4.* [Online] 1958.

83. **Athoo, Tasnim, Aleck Ostry.** *The One Best Way?: Breastfeeding History, Politics, and Policy in Canada.* Apr : Wilfrid Laurier Univ. Press, 2011.

84. vitamindcouncil.org. *https://www.vitamindcouncil.org/a-look-back-at-2012-a-few-key-randomized-controlled-trials/.* [Online] vitamin d council, 2012.

85. Antibiotics. *Wikipedia, the Free Encyclopedia.* [Online] https://en.wikipedia.org/wiki/Antibiotics.

86. Kleist, T. "Bee Navigation: The Eyes Have It." *Science News 130.14 (1986): 214.*

87. https://www.ncbi.nlm.nih.gov/pmc/articles/PMC3897598/. *Spina C, Tangpricha V, Yao M, Zhou W, Wolfe MM, Maehr H, et al. Colon cancer and solar ultraviolet B radiation and prevention and treatment of colon cancer in mice with vitamin D and its Gemini analogs. J Steroid Biochem Mol Biol. 2005;97:111–20. doi: 10.* [Online]

88. https://www.ncbi.nlm.nih.gov/pmc/articles/PMC3897598/. *Ladizesky M, Lu Z, Oliveri B, San Roman N, Diaz S, Holick MF, et al. Solar ultraviolet B radiation and photoproduction of vitamin D3 in central and southern areas of Argentina. J Bone Miner Res. 1995;10:545–9. doi: 10.1002/jbmr.5650100406.* [Online]

89. **Immunology, and Allergy Clinics of North America.** Science Direct. *http://www.sciencedirect.com/science/article/pii/S0889856110000433.* [Online] Aug 2010.

90. **Barton .** The Search for Health in the high Alps of Switzerland. [Online] 2013. http://www.ruralhistory2013.org/papers/4.2.3._Barton.pdf.

91. **Celarier, Herman and.** http://onlinelibrary.wiley.com/doi/10.1029/97JD02074/abstract. *Earth surface reflectivity climatology at 340–380 nm from TOMS data.* [Online] 1997.

92. Ultraviolet Radiation: How it affects Life on Earth. *NASA Earth observatory.* [Online] https://earthobservatory.nasa.gov/Features/UVB/uvb_radiation3.php.

93. https://www.ncbi.nlm.nih.gov/pmc/articles/PMC3897598/. *Luxwolda MF, Kuipers RS, Kema IP, Dijck-Brouwer DA, Muskiet FAJ. Traditionally living populations in East Africa have a mean serum 25-hydroxyvitamin D concentration of 115 nmol/l. Br J Nutr. 2012;108:1557–61. doi: 10.1017/S0007114511007161.* [Online]

94. **Cichorek, Mirosława.** *Skin melanocytes: biology and development.* https://www.ncbi.nlm.nih.gov/pmc/articles/PMC3834696/, 2020.

95. https://www.ncbi.nlm.nih.gov/pmc/articles/PMC3897598/. Matsuoka LY, Wortsman J, Hanifan N, Holick MF. Chronic sunscreen use decreases circulating concentrations of 25-hydroxyvitamin D. A preliminary study. Arch Dermatol. 1988;124:1802–4. doi: 10.1001/archderm.1988.01670120018003,

96. Matsuoka LY, Ide L, Wortsman J, MacLaughlin JA, Holick MF. Sunscreens suppress cutaneous vitamin D3 synthesis. J Clin Endocrinol Metab. 1987;64:1165–8. doi: 10.1210/jcem-64-6-1165. https://www.ncbi.nlm.nih.gov/pmc/articles/PMC3897598/,

97. **Wacker, Matthias, Michael Hollick.** Sunlight and Vitamin D A global perspective for health. *PMC.* [Online] Jan 2013. https://www.ncbi.nlm.nih.gov/pmc/articles/PMC3897598/.

98. *http://drholick.com/ und https://www.youtube.com/watch?v=u7FnJRxUAzI.*

99. *Carlberg C, Seuter S, Heikkinen S. The first genome-wide view of vitamin D receptor locations and their mechanistic implications. Anticancer Res. 2012 Jan;32(1):271-82. Review. PubMed PMID: 22213316.*

100. **Irfete S. Fetahu, Julia Höbaus, and Enikő Kállay*.** Vitamin D and the epigenome. *PMC.* [Online] May 2014. https://www.ncbi.nlm.nih.gov/pmc/articles/PMC4010791/.

101. **Maseeh, Rathish Nair and Arun.** https://www.ncbi.nlm.nih.gov/pmc/articles/PMC3356951/. *Vitamin D: The "sunshine" vitamin.* [Online] 2012.

102. **Silvagno F1, De Vivo E, Attanasio A, Gallo V, Mazzucco G, Pescarmona G.** Mitochondrial localization of vitamin D receptor in human platelets and differentiated megakaryocytes. *PubMed.* [Online] Jan 2010. https://www.ncbi.nlm.nih.gov/pubmed/20107497.

103. **Yanping Lin, a John L. Ubels,b Mark P. Schotanus,b Zhaohong Yin,c Victorina Pintea,c Bruce D. Hammock,a and Mitchell A. Watskyc.** Enhancement of Vitamin D Metabolites in the Eye following Vitamin D3 Supplementation and UV-B Irradiation. *PMC.* [Online] Oct 2013. https://www.ncbi.nlm.nih.gov/pmc/articles/PMC3572765/.

104. *Grant WB. The prevalence of multiple sclerosis in 3 US communities: the role of vitamin D. Prev Chronic Dis. 2010;7:A89–, author reply A90.* https://www.ncbi.nlm.nih.gov/pmc/articles/PMC3897598/ : s.n.

105. **Bhalla AK, Amento EP, Clemens TL, Holick MF, Krane SM.** Specific high-affinity receptors for 1,25-dihydroxyvitamin D3 in human peripheral blood mononuclear cells: presence in monocytes and induction in T lymphocytes following activation. J Clin Endocrinol . *PubMed.* [Online] 1983. https://www.ncbi.nlm.nih.gov/pubmed/6313738.

106. *https://www.ncbi.nlm.nih.gov/pmc/articles/PMC3897598/.*

107. **Adams JS, Gacad MA.** Characterization of 1 alpha-hydroxylation of vitamin D3 sterols by cultured alveolar macrophages from patients with sarcoidosis. J Exp Med. *PubMed.* [Online] 1985. https://www.ncbi.nlm.nih.gov/pubmed/3838552.

108. *Schultz M, Butt AG. Is the north to south gradient in inflammatory bowel disease a global phenomenon? Expert Rev Gastroenterol Hepatol. 2012;6:445–7. doi: 10.1586/egh.12.31.* https://www.ncbi.nlm.nih.gov/pmc/articles/PMC3897598/ : s.n.

109. *Wacker M, Holick MF. Vitamin D - effects on skeletal and extraskeletal health and the need for supplementation. Nutrients. 2013;5:111–48. doi: 10.3390/nu5010111.* https://www.ncbi.nlm.nih.gov/pmc/articles/PMC3897598/ : s.n.

110. **Baker AR, McDonnell DP, Hughes M, et al.** Cloning and expression of full-length cDNA encoding human vitamin D receptor. Proc Natl Acad Sci U S A. . *PubMed.* [Online] 1988. https://www.ncbi.nlm.nih.gov/pubmed/2835767.

111. *Grant WB. Ecological studies of the UVB-vitamin D-cancer hypothesis. Anticancer Res. 2012;32:223–36.* https://www.ncbi.nlm.nih.gov/pmc/articles/PMC3897598/ : s.n.

112. **Wesley, J. Pike, Ph.D. and Mark B. Meyer, Ph.D.** The Vitamin D Receptor: New Paradigms for the Regulation of Gene Expression by 1,25-Dihydroxyvitamin D3. *PMC.* [Online] Jan 2011. https://www.ncbi.nlm.nih.gov/pmc/articles/PMC2879406/.

113. **Sean T. Corbetta, Oya Hillb, Ajay K. Nangiaa, , .** Vitamin D receptor found in human sperm. *Science Direct.* [Online] Dec 2006. http://www.sciencedirect.com/science/article/pii/S0090429506021339.

114. **Shaffer PL1, Gewirth DT.** Vitamin D receptor-DNA interactions. *PubMed.* [Online] https://www.ncbi.nlm.nih.gov/pubmed/15193458.

115. **Holick, Michael F., Neil C. Binkley, Heike A. Bischoff-Ferrari, Catherine M. Gordon, David A. Hanley, Robert P. Heaney, M. Hassan Murad, and Connie M. Weaver.** *Evaluation, Treatment, and Prevention of Vitamin D Deficiency: an Endocrine Society Clinical Practice Guideline - .* The Journal of Clinical Endocrinology & Metabolism : s.n., 2011.

116. **GARLAND, CEDRIC F. , CHRISTINE B. FRENCH, LEO L. BAGGERLY and ROBERT P. HEANEY.** *Vitamin D Supplement Doses and Serum 25-Hydroxyvitamin.* ANTICANCER RESEARCH 31: 617-622 (2011) : s.n.

117. **DP, Trivedi.** *Trivedi DP, Doll R, Khaw KT. Effect of four monthly oral vitamin D3 (cholecalciferol) supplementationon fractures and mortality in men and women living in the community: randomised double blind controlled trial. BMJ. Mar 1;326 (7387):469. 2003.* BMJ. Mar 1;326 (7387):469. 2003 : s.n., 2003.

118. **Grassroots.** *http://www.vitamindwiki.com/Chart+of+Vitamin+D+levels+vs+disease+-+Grassroots+Health+June+2013.* [Online]

119. **Alberts, Bruce, Alexander Johnson, Julian Lewis, Martin Raff, Keith Roberts, and Peter Walter.** *Molecular Biology of the Cell, 4th edition.* New York : Garland Science, 2002. ISBN-10: 0-8153-3218-1ISBN-10: 0-8153-4072-9.

120. **Ignacio Gonzalez-Suarez,1 Abena B Redwood,1 David A Grotsky,1 Martin A Neumann,1 Emily H-Y Cheng,2 Colin L Stewart,3 Adriana Dusso,1,4 and Susana Gonzaloa,1.** A new pathway that regulates 53BP1 stability implicates Cathepsin L and vitamin D in DNA repair. *NCBI.* [Online] Aug 2011. https://www.ncbi.nlm.nih.gov/pmc/articles/PMC3160650/.

121. **Aranow, Cynthia.** Vitamin D and the Immune System. *NCBI.* [Online] Aug 2011. https://www.ncbi.nlm.nih.gov/pmc/articles/PMC3166406/.

122. **Diane L. Kamen and Vin Tangprichacorresponding author.** Williams C. On the use and administration of cod-liver oil in pulmonary consumption. *NCBI.* [Online] Feb 2010. https://www.ncbi.nlm.nih.gov/pmc/articles/PMC2861286/.

123. *Quand la Suisse luttait contre la tuberculose. http://www.rts.ch/archives/tv/culture/calendrier-de-l-histoire/5834254-guerir-grace-au-soleil.html.* [Online] 10 1963.

124. Treatments of Tuberculosis. *CANADA's ROLE in fighting tuberculosis.* [Online] http://sct.poumon.ca/tb/tbhistory/treatment/heliotherapy.html.

125. Neue Züricher Zeitung Vergessener Alpenmediziner aus dem Engadin. *http://www.nzz.ch/vergessener-alpenmediziner-aus-dem-engadin-1.10775400*. [Online] 6 1, 2011.

126. **Hobsay, R.A.** Sunlight Therapy and Solar Architecture. [Online] 1997. https://www.cambridge.org/core/services/aop-cambridge-core/content/view/8A22D374344BE18218FFF37F46591C82/S0025727300063043a.pdf/div-class-title-sunlight-therapy-and-solar-architecture-div.pdf.

127. **Moritz, Andreas.** *Heal Yourself with Sunlight.* U.S.A. : Ener-chi Wellness Press, 2005. ISBN: 978-0-9792757-3-9.

128. **sharecare.** How do the various T cells function in the immune system? *sharecare.* [Online] https://www.sharecare.com/health/immune-lymphatic-system-health/how-t-cells-function-immune.

129. **Komaroff, Dr. Anthony.** How do the various T cells function in the immune system? *sharecare.* [Online] https://www.sharecare.com/health/immune-lymphatic-system-health/how-t-cells-function-immune.

130. **Lehmann B1, Rudolph T, Pietzsch J, Meurer M.** Conversion of vitamin D3 to 1alpha,25-dihydroxyvitamin D3 in human skin equivalents. *NCBI.* [Online] Apr 9, 2000. https://www.ncbi.nlm.nih.gov/pmc/articles/PMC2861286/.

131. Queen Mary University of London. *http://www.qmul.ac.uk/media/news/items/smd/180791.html*. [Online] Sep 2016.

132. Cochrane Review. *http://www.cochrane.org/news/high-quality-evidence-suggests-vitamin-d-can-reduce-asthma-attacks*. [Online] 2016.

133. **Martineau AR, Cates CJ, Urashima M, Jensen M, Griffiths AP, Nurmatov U, Sheikh A, Griffiths CJ. .** High quality evidence suggests Vitamin D can reduce asthma attacks. *Cochrane trusted evidence.* [Online] 2016. http://www.cochrane.org/news/high-quality-evidence-suggests-vitamin-d-can-reduce-asthma-attacks.

134. *Study of serum vitamin D level in adult patientes with bronchial asthma.* http://www.sciencedirect.com/science/article/pii/S0422763816302485, s.l. : Egyption Journal of Chest Diseases and Tuberculosis, 1 11, 2017.

135. VitaminDwiki. *http://www.vitamindwiki.com/The+worse+the+bronchial+asthma%2C+the+lower+the+vitamin+D+%E2%80%93+Jan+2017*. [Online] 1 11, 2017.

136. **Cannell JJ1, Vieth R, Umhau JC, Holick MF, Grant WB, Madronich S, Garland CF, Giovannucci E.** Epidemic influenza and vitamin D. *PubMed.* [Online] Dec 2006. https://www.ncbi.nlm.nih.gov/pubmed/16959053.

137. **Edlich RF, Mason SS, Dahlstrom JJ, Swainston E, Long WB 3rd, Gubler K.** Pandemic preparedness for swine flu influenza in the United States. *PubMed.* [Online] 2009. https://www.ncbi.nlm.nih.gov/pubmed/20102323.

138. **Mitsuyoshi Urashima, Hidetoshi Mezawa, Miki Noya and Carlos A. Camargo.** Effect of Vitamin D Supplement on Influenza A Illness during the 2009 H1N1 Pandemic: A Randomized Controlled Trial. *VitaminDWiki.* [Online] Jul 2014. http://www.vitamindwiki.com/Influenza+A%3A+5X+reduction+in+first+month+%28only%29+with+2%2C000+IU+of+vitamin+D%E2%80%93+RCT+July+2014.

139. **Canell, JJ, et al.** Randomized trial of vitamin D supplementation to prevent seasonal influenza A in schoolchildren1,2,3. *The American Journal of Clinical Nutrition.* [Online] 2010. http://ajcn.nutrition.org/content/91/5/1255.full.

140. **Torres, Marco.** Vitamin D Proven More Effective Than Both Anti-Viral Drugs and Vaccines At Preventing The Flu. *PreventDisease.* [Online] Oct 2013. https://preventdisease.com/news/13/102213_Vitamin-D-Proven-More-Effective-Anti-Viral-Drugs-Vaccines-Preventing-Flu.shtml.

141. **Milo F. Vassallo, MD, PhD, Carlos A. Camargo Jr.** Potential mechanisms for the hypothesized link between sunshine, vitamin D, and food allergy in children. [Online] The journal of Allergy and clinical Immunology, Aug 2010. http://www.jacionline.org/article/S0091-6749(10)00968-1/fulltext.

142. *The link between serum vitamin D level, sensitization to food allergens, and the severity of atopic dermatitis in infancy.* https://www.ncbi.nlm.nih.gov/pubmed/25108543, Oct 2014.

143. The Link between Serum Vitamin D Level, Sensitization to Food Allergens, and the Severity of Atopic Dermatitis in Infancy. *Researchgate.* [Online] https://www.researchgate.net/publication/264628965_The_Link_between_Serum_Vitamin_D_Level_Sensitization_to_Food_Allergens_and_the_Severity_of_Atopic_Dermatitis_in_Infancy.

144. **Feuille, Elizabeth J., Anna H. Nowak-Węgrzyn.** Vitamin D Insufficiency Is Associated With Challenge-Proven Food Allergy in Infants. *http://pediatrics.aappublications.org/content/132/Supplement_1/S7.short#*. [Online] Oct 2013.

145. **Nkemcho Ojeh, 1 Irena Pastar,2 Marjana Tomic-Canic,2 and Olivera Stojadinovic2,.** Stem Cells in Skin Regeneration, Wound Healing, and Their Clinical Applications. *PMC.* [Online] Oct 2015. https://www.ncbi.nlm.nih.gov/pmc/articles/PMC4632811/.

146. **Bikle, Daniel David .** Role of vitamin D and calcium signaling in wound healing . *Grantome.* [Online] http://grantome.com/grant/NIH/I01-BX001066-04.

147. **Bikle, Daniel David .** Role of vitamin D and calcium signaling in wound healing. *National Institutes of Health.* [Online] 2014. http://grantome.com/grant/NIH/I01-BX001066-04.

148. **Whitney P Bowecorresponding author1 and Alan C Logancorresponding author2.** Acne vulgaris, probiotics and the gut-brain-skin axis - back to the future? *NCBI.* [Online] 2011. https://www.ncbi.nlm.nih.gov/pmc/articles/PMC3038963/.

149. Vitamin D supplements significantly improve symptoms of winter-related atopic dermatitis in children. *Massachusets General Hospital.* [Online] Oct 2014. http://www.massgeneral.org/about/pressrelease.aspx?id=1746.

150. **PMC.** *Vitamin D in Atopic Dermatitis, Asthma and Allergic Diseases.* https://www.ncbi.nlm.nih.gov/pmc/articles/PMC2914320/ : s.n., 2011.

151. **Hegazy, Wedad Z. Mostafa⬚ and Rehab A.** Vitamin D and the skin: Focus on a complex relationship: A review. *PubMed.* [Online] Nov 2015. https://www.ncbi.nlm.nih.gov/pmc/articles/PMC4642156/.

152. **Helden, Dr. Raimund.** Vitamindelta. [Online] 2015. http://www.vitamindelta.de/.

153. **Hata, Tissa R. MD, Paul Kotol, BS, Michelle Jackson, MD, Meggie Nguyen, BS, Aimee Paik, MD, Don Udall, MD, Kimi Kanada, BS, Kenshi Yamasaki, MD, Phd, Doru Alexandrescu, MD, and Richard L. Gallo, MD, PhD.** Administration of oral vitamin D induces cathelicidin production in atopic individuals. *PMC.* [Online] Oct 2008. https://www.ncbi.nlm.nih.gov/pmc/articles/PMC2659525/.

154. *Morimoto S, Yoshikawa K, Kozuka T et al: An open study of vitamin D3 treatment in psoriasis vulgaris. Br J Dermatol; 115(4):421-429.* 1986.

155. *J Intern Med. Apr;253(4):439-46. 2003.*

156. **Reichrath, Jörg (Ed.).** http://www.springer.com/us/book/9781493904365. s.l. : Springer, 2014. ISBN 978-1-4939-0437-2.

157. **Helden, Raimund von, MD.** Was können wir gegen Strahlenschäden tun? Vitamin D als natürliches Zellschutz-System ! *Vitamin D Service.* [Online] 2016. https://www.vitamindservice.de/was-k%C3%B6nnen-wir-gegen-strahlensch%C3%A4den-tun-vitamin-d-als-nat%C3%BCrliches-zellschutz-system.

158. **Naghii MR1.** Sulfur mustard intoxication, oxidative stress, and antioxidants. *PubMed.* [Online] Jul 2002. https://www.ncbi.nlm.nih.gov/pubmed/12125850.

159. **Das LM1, Binko AM1, Traylor ZP1, Duesler LR1, Dynda SM1, Debanne S2, Lu KQ3.** Early indicators of survival following exposure to mustard gas: Protective role of 25(OH)D. [Online] Mar 2016. https://www.ncbi.nlm.nih.gov/pubmed/26940683.

160. **Shirazi HA1, Rasouli J1, Ciric B1, Rostami A1, Zhang GX2.** 1,25-Dihydroxyvitamin D3 enhances neural stem cell proliferation and oligodendrocyte differentiation. *PubMed.* [Online] Apr 2015. https://www.ncbi.nlm.nih.gov/pubmed/25681066.

161. **Metabolism, Trends in Endocrinology &.** Garcion, Emmanuel, et al. New clues about vitamin D functions in the nervous system. , 2002, 13. Jg., Nr. 3, S. 100-105. *PubMed.* [Online] 2002. https://www.ncbi.nlm.nih.gov/pubmed/11893522.

162. **Garcion, E, Wion-Barbot N, Montero-Menei CN, Berger F, Wion D.** New clues about vitamin D functions in the nervous system. *PubMed.* [Online] https://www.ncbi.nlm.nih.gov/pubmed/11893522.

163. **DeLuca GC1, Kimball SM, Kolasinski J, Ramagopalan SV, Ebers GC.** Review: the role of vitamin D in nervous system health and disease. *PubMed.* [Online] Aug 2013. https://www.ncbi.nlm.nih.gov/pubmed/23336971.

164. Depression. *World Health Organization.* [Online] 2017. http://www.who.int/mediacentre/factsheets/fs369/en/.

165. **Jordanes.** *The Origin and Deeds of the Goths. Mierow C.C., editor. Princeton University Press; Princeton, NJ, USA:.* https://www.ncbi.nlm.nih.gov/pmc/articles/PMC4011048/ : s.n., 2012. pp. 19–21.

166. **Hoogendijk WJ1, Lips P, Dik MG, Deeg DJ, Beekman AT, Penninx BW.** Depression is associated with decreased 25-hydroxyvitamin D and increased parathyroid hormone levels in older adults. *PubMed.* [Online] May 2008. https://www.ncbi.nlm.nih.gov/pubmed/18458202.

167. **Bertone-Johnson .** Vitamin D and the occurrence of depression: causal association or circumstantial evidence? *PubMed.* [Online] Aug 2009. https://www.ncbi.nlm.nih.gov/pubmed/19674344.

168. **Ganji V., Milone C., Cody M., McCarty F., Wang Y.T.** Serum Vitamin D concentrations are related to depression in young adult US population: The Third National Health and Nutrition Examination Survey. . *PubMed.* [Online] 2010. https://www.ncbi.nlm.nih.gov/pmc/articles/PMC4011048/.

169. **Umhau J.C., George D.T., Heaney R.P., Lewis M.D., Ursano R.J. Low Vitamin D status and suicide: A case-control study of active duty military service members. PLoS One. 2013 and 8:e51543.** Low Vitamin D status and suicide: A case-control study of active duty military service members. . *PubMed.* [Online] 2013. https://www.ncbi.nlm.nih.gov/pmc/articles/PMC4011048/.

170. Seasonal affective disorder: It's not what you think. *The Psychiatry Letter.* [Online] http://www.psychiatryletter.org/SAD2.html.

171. **Boerman R, Cohen D, Schulte PF, Nugter A.** Prevalence of Vitamin D Deficiency in Adult Outpatients With Bipolar Disorder or Schizophrenia. *PubMed.* [Online] Dec 2016. https://www.ncbi.nlm.nih.gov/pubmed/27662458.

172. **Vaziri F1, Nasiri S2, Tavana Z3, Dabbaghmanesh MH4, Sharif F5, Jafari P6.** Perinatal depression decreased 40 percent with just a few weeks of 2,000 IU of vitamin D – RCT Aug 2016. *VitaminDWiki.* [Online] Aug 20, 2016. http://www.vitamindwiki.com/Perinatal+depression+decreased+40+percent+with+just+a+few+weeks+of+2%2C000+IU+of+vitamin+D+%E2%80%93+RCT+Aug+2016.

173. **Sturges, M.** Low vitamin D status associated with gastric dysmotility in newly diagnosed Parkinson's patients. *Vitamin D Council.* [Online] June23 2016. https://www.vitamindcouncil.org/low-vitamin-d-status-associated-with-gastric-dysmotility-in-newly-diagnosed-parkinsons-patients/.

174. **Peterson, Amie L.** A Review of Vitamin D and Parkinson's Disease. *Resesarch Gate.* [Online] May 2014. https://www.researchgate.net/publication/260558617_A_Review_of_Vitamin_D_and_Parkinson%27s_Disease.

175. **Oshiro, Rebeccca.** An overview on current evidence on vitamin D and brain disorders. *Vitamin D Council.* [Online] Sep 2013. https://www.vitamindcouncil.org/an-overview-on-current-evidence-on-vitamin-d-and-brain-disorders/.

176. **Rimmelzwaan LM1, van Schoor NM2, Lips P1, Berendse HW3, Eekhoff EM1.** Systematic Review of the Relationship between Vitamin D and Parkinson's Disease. *PubMed.* [Online] June 2016. https://www.ncbi.nlm.nih.gov/pubmed/26756741.

177. **Cebulla, Brant.** New trial says, vitamin D prevents progression and deterioration of Parkinson's Disease. *Vitamin D Council.* [Online] March 2013. https://www.vitamindcouncil.org/new-trial-says-vitamin-d-prevents-progression-and-deterioration-of-parkinsons-disease/.

178. What is dementia? [Online] http://www.alzheimers.org.uk/info/20007/types_of_dementia/1/what_is_dementia.

179. **Beilharz, Jessica E. , Jayanthi Maniam, and Margaret J. Morris*.** Diet-Induced Cognitive Deficits: The Role of Fat and Sugar, Potential Mechanisms and Nutritional Interventions. *PMC.* [Online] Aug 2015. https://www.ncbi.nlm.nih.gov/pmc/articles/PMC4555146/.

180. Lack of vitamin D linked to higher dementia risk. *yahoo news.* [Online] Aug 2014. Lack of vitamin D linked to higher dementia risk.

181. **Sauer, Alissa.** Link Found between Vitamin D Deficiency and Dementia. *alzheimers.net.* [Online] Oct 2015. http://www.alzheimers.net/8-27-14-vitamin-d-and-dementia/.

182. How many people are affected by autism spectrum disorder (ASD)? *Centers for Disease Control and prevention.* [Online] https://www.cdc.gov/ncbddd/autism/data.html.

183. **Tovey, Amber.** Vitamin D supplementation improves autism in children, according to new study. *Vitamin D Council.* [Online] Dec 7, 2016. https://www.vitamindcouncil.org/vitamin-d-supplementation-improves-autism-in-children-according-to-new-study/.

184. **Saad K1, Abdel-Rahman AA2, Elserogy YM2, Al-Atram AA3, El-Houfey AA4, Othman HA5, Bjørklund G6, Jia F7, Urbina MA8,9, Abo-Elela MG10, Ahmad FA1, Abd El-Baseer KA10, Ahmed AE10, Abdel-Salam AM11.** Randomized controlled trial of vitamin D supplementation in children with autism spectrum disorder. *PubMed.* [Online] Nov 21, 2016. https://www.ncbi.nlm.nih.gov/pubmed/27868194.

185. Epilepsy. *World Health Organization.* [Online] 2017. http://www.who.int/mediacentre/factsheets/fs999/en/.

186. **Kevin Pendo and Christopher M. DeGiorgio, MD1.** Epilepsy appears to be treated by Vitamin D (starting 5,000 IU RCT) – Dec 2016. [Online] 2016. http://www.vitamindwiki.com/Idiopathic+Epileptic+children+have+low+levels+of+vitamin+D+%E2%80%93+Oct+2015#Epilepsy_appears_to_be_treated_by_Vitamin_D_starting_5_000_IU_RCT_Dec_2016.

187. **Holló,András , Zsófia Clemens, and Péter Lakatos.** Epilepsy and Vitamin D. *tandfonline.* [Online] 2014. http://www.tandfonline.com/doi/abs/10.3109/00207454.2013.847836.

188. **May, Epilepsy Behav. 2012 and 11., 24(1):131-3. doi: 10.1016/j.yebeh.2012.03.011. Epub 2012 Apr.** Correction of vitamin D deficiency improves seizure control in epilepsy: a pilot study. *OubMed.* [Online] May 2012. https://www.ncbi.nlm.nih.gov/pubmed/22503468.

189. **Brazier, Yvette.** Low vitamin D and obesity as teenagers may accelerate MS. *Medical News Today .* [Online] Oct 8, 2015. http://www.medicalnewstoday.com/articles/300576.php.

190. **Fitzgerald KC1, Munger KL1, Köchert K2, Arnason BG3, Comi G4, Cook S5, Goodin DS6, Filippi M7, Hartung HP8, Jeffery DR9, O'Connor P10, Suarez G11, Sandbrink R12, Kappos L13, Pohl C14, Ascherio A15.** Association of Vitamin D Levels With Multiple Sclerosis Activity and Progression in Patients Receiving Interferon Beta-1b. *PubMed.* [Online] Dec 2015. https://www.ncbi.nlm.nih.gov/pubmed/26458124.

191. Early stage study shows that vitamin D can promote myelin repair. *Latest MS Research news.* [Online] Dec 2015. https://mssociety.ca/research-news/article/early-stage-study-shows-that-vitamin-d-can-promote-myelin-repair.

192. **Alerie Guzman de la Fuente, Oihana Errea, Peter van Wijngaarden, Ginez A. Gonzalez, Christophe Kerninon, Andrew A. Jarjour, Hilary J. Lewis, Clare A. Jones, Brahim Nait-Oumesmar, Chao Zhao, Jeffrey K. Huang, Charles ffrench-Constant, Robin J.M. Franklin.** Vitamin D receptor–retinoid X receptor heterodimer signaling regulates oligodendrocyte progenitor cell differentiation. *The Rockefeller University Press.* [Online] Dec 2015. http://jcb.rupress.org/content/211/5/975.

193. **Hartung, Hans Peter, Ludwig Kappos, Douglas S. Goodin, Paul O'Connor, Massimo Filippi, Barry Arnason, Giancarlo Comi, Stuart Cook, Douglas Jeffery, John Petkau, Richard White, Timon Bogumil, Karola Beckmann, Brigitte Stemper, Gustavo Su.** Predictors of disease activity in 857 patients with MS treated with interferon beta-1b. *PMC.* [Online] Aug 2015. https://www.ncbi.nlm.nih.gov/pmc/articles/PMC4639578/.

194. **Cannell, John, MD.** Is it sunshine or vitamin D that helps multiple sclerosis (MS) patients? *Vitamin D Council.* [Online] Oct 16, 2015. https://www.vitamindcouncil.org/is-it-sunshine-or-vitamin-d-that-helps-multiple-sclerosis-ms-patients/.

195. Cell-based study reveals that vitamin D can drive the activity of neural stem cells that promote myelin repair. *Latest MS Reserch News.* [Online] Mar 30, 2015. https://mssociety.ca/research-news/article/cell-based-study-reveals-that-vitamin-d-can-drive-the-activity-of-neural-stem-cells-that-promote-myelin-repair.

196. **Funte, de la AG, Errea O, van Wijngaarden P, Gonzalez GA, Kerninon C, Jarjour AA, Lewis HJ, Jones CA, Nait-Oumesmar B, Zhao C, Huang JK, ffrench-Constant C, Franklin RJ.** Vitamin D receptor-retinoid X receptor heterodimer signaling regulates oligodendrocyte progenitor cell differentiation. *PubMed.* [Online] Dec 7, 2015. https://www.ncbi.nlm.nih.gov/pubmed/26644513.

197. Closer look: vitamin D may help protect the brain in MS patients. *vitamindcouncil.* [Online] Nov 30, 2015. ps://www.vitamindcouncil.org/closer-look-vitamin-d-may-help-protect-the-brain-in-ms-patients/.

198. **Mowry EM1, Pelletier D2, Gao Z3, Howell MD3, Zamvil SS4, Waubant E4.** Vitamin D in clinically isolated syndrome: evidence for possible neuroprotection. *PubMed.* [Online] Feb 2016. https://www.ncbi.nlm.nih.gov/pubmed/?term=Vitamin+D+in+clinically+isolated+syndrome%3A+evidence+for+possible+neuroprotection.

199. MS: Epidemiology and Prevalence . [Online] [Cited:]

200. MS: Epidemiology and Prevalence. *library med.utah.* [Online] http://library.med.utah.edu/kw/ms/epidemiology.html.

201. The top 10 causes of death. *World Health Organization.* [Online] Jan 2017. http://www.who.int/mediacentre/factsheets/fs310/en/.

202. **HR, Barthel.** Barthel HR, Scharla SH. *[Benefits beyond the bones -- vitamin D against falls, cancer, hypertension and autoimmune diseases] Dtsch Med Wochenschr. Feb 28;128(9):440-6. [Article in German] 2003.* Med Wochenschr. Feb 28;128(9):440-6 : s.n., 2003.

203. **Carl J. Lavie, MD, John H. Lee, MD and Richard V. Milani, MD.** Vitamin D and Cardiovascular Disease. *Medscape.* [Online] 2011. http://www.medscape.com/viewarticle/750679_8.

204. **Dobnig H1, Pilz S, Scharnagl H, Renner W, Seelhorst U, Wellnitz B, Kinkeldei J, Boehm BO, Weihrauch G, Maerz W.** Independent association of low serum 25-hydroxyvitamin d and 1,25-dihydroxyvitamin d levels with all-cause and cardiovascular mortality. *PubMed.* [Online] Jun 23, 2008. https://www.ncbi.nlm.nih.gov/pubmed/18574092.

205. **Wang TJ, Pencina MJ, Booth SL, Jacques PF, Ingelsson E, Lanier K, Benjamin EJ, D'Agostino RB, Wolf M, Vasan RS.** Vitamin D deficiency and risk of cardiovascular disease. *PubMed.* [Online] Jan 29, 2008. https://www.ncbi.nlm.nih.gov/pubmed/18180395.

206. Zittermann A, Schleithoff SS, Tenderich G, Berthold HK, Korfer R, Stehle P. *Low vitamin D status: a contributing factor in the pathogenesis of congestive heart failure? J Am Coll Cardiol. Jan 1;41(1):105-12. 2003.*

207. **K, Nishio.** Nishio K, Mukae S, Aoki S, Itoh S, Konno N, Ozawa K, Satoh R, Katagiri T. *Congestive heart failure is associated with the rate of bone loss. J Intern Med. Apr;253(4):439-46. 2003.* J Intern Med. Apr;253(4):439-46. 2003 : s.n., 2003.

208. **Burgaz, A., Orsini, N., Larsson, S.C. et al.** *Blood 25-hydroxyvitamin D concentration and hypertension: a meta-analysis.* . Journal of Hypertension, 29, 636-645 : s.n., 2011.

209. **Pittas, A.G., Chung, M., Trikalinos, T. et al.** *Systematic review: Vitamin D and cardiometabolic outcomes.* Annals of Internal Medicine : s.n., 2009.

210. **Stefan Pilz, Andreas Tomaschitz, Winfried Maerz–, Christiane Drechsler, Eberhard Ritz††, Armin Zittermann‡‡, Etienne Cavalier Thomas R. Pieber, Joan M. Lappe, William B. Grant, Michael F. Holick and Jacqueline M. Dekker.** Vitamin D, cardiovascular disease and mortality. *Wiley Online Library.* [Online] Oct 4, 2011. http://onlinelibrary.wiley.com/doi/10.1111/j.1365-2265.2011.04147.x/full.

211. **Pilz, S., Iodice, S., Zittermann, A. et al.** Vitamin D status and mortality risk in chronic kidney disease: a meta-analysis of prospective studies. *PubMed.* [Online] Sep 2011. https://www.ncbi.nlm.nih.gov/pubmed/21636193.

212. **Autier, P. & Gandini, S.** *Vitamin D supplementation and total mortality: a meta-analysis of randomized controlled trials.* . Archives of Internal Medicine, 167, 1730–1737 : s.n., 2007.

213. Clinical Endocrinology . *https://www.meandermc.nl/wps/wcm/connect/www/210ec54a-cfef-41a8-ae2c-717b9d12befe/Vitamin+D,+cardiovascular+disease+and+mortality.pdf?MOD=AJPERES.* [Online] 2011.

214. **Oh, J., Weng, S., Felton, S.K. et al.** *1,25(OH)2 vitamin d inhibits foam cell formation and suppresses macrophage cholesterol.* Circulation 120, 687-698 : s.n., 2009.

215. **Pilz, S., Tomaschitz, A., Drechsler, C. et al.** *Parathyroid hormone level is associated with mortality and cardiovascular events in patients undergoing coronary angiography.* . European Heart Journal : s.n., 2010.

216. **Kalkan GY1, Gür M2, Koyunsever NY1, Şeker T1, Gözükara MY3, Uçar H1, Kaypaklı O1, Baykan AO1, Akyol S1, Türkoğlu C1, Elbasan Z1, Şahin DY1, Çaylı M1.** Serum 25-Hydroxyvitamin D Level and Aortic Intima-Media Thickness in Patients Without Clinical Manifestation of Atherosclerotic Cardiovascular Disease. *PubMed.* [Online] Jul 2015. https://www.ncbi.nlm.nih.gov/pubmed/25130180.

217. **Mandal, Dr. Ananya.** What is metabolism? [Online] http://www.news-medical.net/life-sciences/What-is-Metabolism.aspx.

218. **Saul, Andrew W. .** Vitamin D: Deficiency, Diversity and Dosage. [Online] 2003. http://orthomolecular.org/library/jom/2003/pdf/2003-v18n0304-p194.pdf.

219. **Mayo Clinic Staff.** Osteoporosis. *Mayo Clinic.* [Online] http://www.mayoclinic.org/diseases-conditions/osteoporosis/home/ovc-20207808.

220. **Bouillon, Roger, Tatsuo Suda.** Vitamin D: calcium and bone homeostasis during evolution. *BoneKEyReports.* [Online] 2014. http://www.nature.com/bonekeyreports/2014/140108/bonekey2013214/full/bonekey2013214.html.

221. Dawson-Hughes B, Harris SS, Krall EA, et al. *Effect of calcium and vitamin D supplementation on bone density in men and women 65 years of age or older. N Engl J Med. 337:670-676. 1997.*

222. **Lips P1, van Schoor NM.** The effect of vitamin D on bone and osteoporosis. *PubMed.* [Online] 2011. https://www.ncbi.nlm.nih.gov/pubmed/21872800.

223. **El Asmar, Margueritta 1 Joseph J. Naoum,2 and Elias J. Arbid.** Vitamin K Dependent Proteins and the Role of Vitamin K2 in the Modulation of Vascular Calcification: A Review. *PMC.* [Online] May 2014. https://www.ncbi.nlm.nih.gov/pmc/articles/PMC4052396/.

224. **Bor, EJ1, van den Hoeven-van Kasteel W, Kelder JC, Lems WF.** Prevalence and correction of severe hypovitaminosis D in patients over 50 years with a low-energy fracture. *PubMed.* [Online] Mar 2015. https://www.ncbi.nlm.nih.gov/pubmed/25852112.

225. **DrBicuspid, Staff.** Study: Dentin shows vitamin D deficiency of earlier civilizations. *Dr Biscuspid.com.* [Online] July 2016. http://www.drbicuspid.com/index.aspx?sec=ser&sub=def&pag=dis&ItemID=320064.

226. **Perayil J1, Menon KS2, Kurup S3, Thomas AE4, Fenol A5, Vyloppillil R5, Bhaskar A6, Megha S7.** Influence of Vitamin D & Calcium Supplementation in the Management of Periodontitis. *PubMed.* [Online] Jun 2015. https://www.ncbi.nlm.nih.gov/pubmed/?term=.+Influence+of+Vitamin+D+%26+Calcium+Supplementation+in+the+Management+of+Periodontitis..

227. Peridontal Disease. *Vitamin D Council.* [Online] 2016. https://www.vitamindcouncil.org/health-conditions/periodontal-disease/.

228. **Ekwaru, John Paul, Jennifer D. Zwicker, Michael F. Holick, Edward Giovannucci, Paul J. Veugelers.** The Importance of Body Weight for the Dose Response Relationship of Oral Vitamin D Supplementation and Serum 25-Hydroxyvitamin D in Healthy Volunteers. *VitaminDWiki*. [Online] Nov 2014. John Paul Ekwaru, Jennifer D. Zwicker, Michael F. Holick, Edward Giovannucci, Paul J. Veugelers.

229. **Jacobo Wortsman Matsuoka Lois Y Matsuoka, L.Y Michael F J Wortsman Matsuoka, Lois Y Jacobo, Wortsman Zhiren Lu L Matsuoka TaiC Chen Tai Michael Holick Tai C, Chen Jacobo Lois Y Lu Zhiren Lu Holick Chen, TC Chen, Tai C Tai Chen Tai C Wortsman.** Decreased bioavailability of vitamin D in obesity1,2,3. *American Society for Clinical Nutrition*. [Online] 2000. http://ajcn.nutrition.org/content/72/3/690.full.

230. **LeBlanc ES, Rizzo JH, Pedula KL, Ensrud KE, Cauley J, Hochberg M, Hillier TA and Fractures., Study Of Osteoporotic.** Associations between 25-hydroxyvitamin D and weight gain in elderly women. *VitaminDWiki*. [Online] Dec 2012. http://www.vitamindwiki.com/tiki-index.php?page_id=3551.

231. **Engelman, Corinne.** Vitamin D may block the obesity gene FTO. *VitaminDWiki* . [Online] Feb 2014. http://www.vitamindwiki.com/Vitamin+D+may+block+the+obesity+gene+%28FTO%29+%E2%80%93+Jan+2014.

232. **Bowles, Jeff T.** *The miraculous results of extremely high doses of the sunshine hormone vitamine D.* Sep : CreateSpace Independent Publishing Platform; Auflage: 1 (2. September 2013), 2013. ISBN-13: 978-1491243824.

233. Overall Numbers, Diabetes and Prediabetes. *American Diabetes Association*. [Online] 2012. http://www.diabetes.org/diabetes-basics/statistics/?referrer=https://www.google.ch/.

234. Diabetes. *World Health Organization*. [Online] 2016. http://www.who.int/mediacentre/factsheets/fs312/en/.

235. **BJ1., Boucher.** Vitamin D insufficiency and diabetes risks. *PubMed*. [Online] Jan 2011. https://www.ncbi.nlm.nih.gov/pubmed/20795936.

236. **Asians., Glucose intolerance and impairment of insulin secretion in relation to vitamin D deficiency in east London.** Glucose intolerance and impairment of insulin secretion in relation to vitamin D deficiency in east London Asians. *PubMed*. [Online] Oct 1995. https://www.ncbi.nlm.nih.gov/pubmed/8690178.

237. **Seyed A. Hoseini, Ashraf Aminorroaya, Bijan Iraj, and Massoud Amini.** The effects of oral vitamin D on insulin resistance in pre-diabetic patients. [Online] Jan 2013. https://www.ncbi.nlm.nih.gov/pmc/articles/PMC3719226/.

238. **Parildar H,Cigerli O, Unal DA, Gulmez O, and Demirag NG.** The impact of Vitamin D Replacement on Glucose Metabolism. *PMC*. [Online] Nov 2013. https://www.ncbi.nlm.nih.gov/pmc/articles/PMC3905396/.

239. **Mercola, MD.** The Relationship Between Vitamin D and Insulin Resistance. *Mercola*. [Online] Jun 29, 2016. http://articles.mercola.com/sites/articles/archive/2016/06/29/vitamin-d-insulin-resistance.aspx.

240. **Mercola, Dr.** The Relationship Between Vitamin D and Insulin Resistance. *Mercola*. [Online] June 29, 2016. http://articles.mercola.com/sites/articles/archive/2016/06/29/vitamin-d-insulin-resistance.aspx.

241. **Afsaneh TalaeiEmail author, Mahnaz Mohamadi and Zahra Adgi.** The effect of vitamin D on insulin resistance in patients with type 2 diabetes. *Diabetology & Metabolic Syndrome*. [Online] 2013. https://dmsjournal.biomedcentral.com/articles/10.1186/1758-5996-5-8.

242. **Ekatha Ann John.** Diabetes in young goes up four-fold: Experts. *The Times of India*. [Online] Nov 2016. http://timesofindia.indiatimes.com/city/chennai/Diabetes-in-young-goes-up-four-fold-Experts/articleshow/55405843.cms.

243. **Lavie, Carl MD, , John H. Lee, MD, Richard V. Milani, MD.** Vitamin D and Cardiovascular Disease : Will It Live Up to its Hype? *Science Direct*. [Online] Oct 2011. http://www.sciencedirect.com/science/article/pii/S0735109711026489.

244. *Mathieu C et al. Prevention of autoimmune diabetes in NOD mice by dihydroxyvitamin D3. Diabetology, v. 37, p. 552-558. 1994.*

245. **Prue H. Hart, Shelley Gorman & John J. Finlay-Jones.** Modulation of the immune system by UV radiation: more than just the effects of vitamin D? *Nature reviews IMMUNOLOGY*. [Online] Sep 2011. http://www.nature.com/nri/journal/v11/n9/full/nri3045.html.

246. **Manila Kaushal and Navneet Magon1.** Vitamin D in pregnancy: A metabolic outlook. *PMC*. [Online] Jan-Feb 2013. https://www.ncbi.nlm.nih.gov/pmc/articles/PMC3659910/.

247. **Zhang C1, Qiu C, Hu FB, David RM, van Dam RM, Bralley A, Williams MA.** Maternal plasma 25-hydroxyvitamin D concentrations and the risk for gestational diabetes mellitus. *PubMed*. [Online] Nov 18, 2008. https://www.ncbi.nlm.nih.gov/pubmed/19015731.

248. **Helden, Dr. von Raimund.** Fussprobleme durch Vitamin D Mangel . *Vitamindelta.de*. [Online] 2014. http://www.vitamindelta.de/faq-frage-antwort/15-fragen-aus-der-praxis/83-fussprobleme-durch-vitamin-d-mangel.html.

249. **Tiwari S1, Pratyush DD, Gupta B, Dwivedi A, Chaudhary S, Rayicherla RK, Gupta SK, Singh SK.** Prevalence and severity of vitamin D deficiency in patients with diabetic foot infection. *PubMed*. [Online] Apr 2012. https://www.ncbi.nlm.nih.gov/pubmed/22715859.

250. **Masterjohn, Chris.** Vitamin D is Synthesized From Cholesterol and Found in Cholesterol-Rich Foods. *Cholesterol and Health*. [Online] May 25, 2006. http://www.cholesterol-and-health.com/Vitamin-D.html.

251. **Schaefer, Anna and Kathryn Watson.** What's the Relationship Between Vitamin D and Cholesterol? *Health Line*. [Online] Mar 2016. http://www.healthline.com/health/high-cholesterol/vitamin-d-relationship.

252. **Tovey, Amber.** Clinical trial finds vitamin D supplementation increases "good" cholesterol in children. *Vitamin D Council*. [Online] Oct 2016. https://www.vitamindcouncil.org/clinical-trial-finds-vitamin-d-supplementation-increases-good-cholesterol-in-children/.

253. **Garland, Dr. Cedric.** Vitamin D & Premenopausal Breast Cancer – Deficiency Increases Risk. *GrassrootsHealth*. [Online] http://www.grassrootshealth.net/garlandbctranscription.

254. **Paddock, Catharine PhD.** Cancer risk falls with higher levels of vitamin D. *Medical News Today.* [Online] Apr 8, 2016. http://www.medicalnewstoday.com/articles/308834.php.

255. **Adams, Mike.** New research shows vitamin D slashes risk of cancers by 77 percent; cancer industry refuses to support cancer prevention. *Natural News.* [Online] June 8, 2007. http://www.naturalnews.com/021892.html.

256. **Li M1, Chen P, Li J, Chu R, Xie D, Wang H.** Review: the impacts of circulating 25-hydroxyvitamin D levels on cancer patient outcomes: a systematic review and meta-analysis. *PubMed.* [Online] Apr 2014. https://www.ncbi.nlm.nih.gov/pubmed/24780061.

257. **http://journals.plos.org/plosone/article?id=10.1371/journal.pone.0152441.** Serum 25-Hydroxyvitamin D Concentrations ≥40 ng/ml Are Associated with >65% Lower Cancer Risk: Pooled Analysis of Randomized Trial and Prospective Cohort Study. *PLOS ONE.* [Online] Apr 6, 2016. http://journals.plos.org/plosone/article?id=10.1371/journal.pone.0152441.

258. **WB1., Grant.** Ecological studies of the UVB-vitamin D-cancer hypothesis. *PubMed.* [Online] Jan 2012. https://www.ncbi.nlm.nih.gov/pubmed/22213311.

259. **Yaw A. Nyame, Adam B. Murphy, Diana K. Bowen, Gregory Jordan, Ken Batai, Michael Dixon, Courtney M.P. Hollowell, Stephanie Kielb...** Associations Between Serum Vitamin D and Adverse Pathology in Men Undergoing Radical Prostatectomy. *Journal of clinical oncology.* [Online] Apr 2016. http://ascopubs.org/doi/abs/10.1200/JCO.2015.65.1463.

260. **Adam B. Murphy, Yaw Nyame, Iman K. Martin, William J. Catalona, Courtney M.P. Hollowell, Robert B. Nadler, James M. Kozlowski, Kent T. Perry, Andre Kajdacsy-Balla and Rick Kittles.** Vitamin D Deficiency Predicts Prostate Biopsy Outcomes. *Clinical Cancer Research.* [Online] May 2014. http://clincancerres.aacrjournals.org/content/20/9/2289.

261. **Garnick, Marc B. M.D.,.** 2017 Annual Report on Prostate Diseases. *Harvard Health Publication.* [Online] 2017. http://www.health.harvard.edu/special-health-reports/2014-annual-report-on-prostate-diseases.

262. **Abdollahi A, Ali-Bakhshi A, Farahani Z.** Concentration Study of High Sensitive C - reactive Protein and some Serum Trace Elements in Patients with Benign and Malignant Breast Tumor. *PubMed.* [Online] https://www.ncbi.nlm.nih.gov/pubmed/26865928.

263. Low vitamin D levels - Breast cancer. *Breast Cancer Org.* [Online] 2014. http://www.breastcancer.org/risk/factors/low_vit_d.

264. Breast cancer. *Vitamin D council.* [Online] Oct. There is growing evidence that solar UVB reduces the risk of breast and other cancers. People who live in the more sunny regions of low to mid-latitude countries have lower breast cancer incidence and/or mortality rates than those living in the higher lat.

265. **Lowe LC1, Guy M, Mansi JL, Peckitt C, Bliss J, Wilson RG, Colston KW.** Plasma 25-hydroxy vitamin D concentrations, vitamin D receptor genotype and breast cancer risk in a UK Caucasian population. *PubMed.* [Online] Apr 14, 2005. https://www.ncbi.nlm.nih.gov/pubmed/15911240.

266. **Arul Vijaya Vani S1, Ananthanarayanan PH2, Kadambari D3, Harichandrakumar KT4, Niranjjan R5, Nandeesha H2.** Effects of vitamin D and calcium supplementation on side effects profile in patients of breast cancer treated with letrozole. *PubMed.* [Online] Aug 2016. Clin Chim Acta. 2016 Aug 1;459:53-6. doi: 10.1016/j.cca.2016.05.020. Epub 2016 May 21..

267. Low Vitamin D Levels. *Breastcancer.org.* [Online] http://www.breastcancer.org/risk/factors/low_vit_d.

268. Pancreas Cancer news. *Medical News Today.* [Online] http://www.medicalnewstoday.com/categories/pancreatic-cancer.

269. **Chiang KC1, Chen TC.** Vitamin D for the prevention and treatment of pancreatic cancer. *PubMed.* [Online] Jul 2009. https://www.ncbi.nlm.nih.gov/pubmed/19610135?dopt=Citation.

270. **Chen Yuan, Zhi Rong Qian, Ana Babic, Vicente Morales-Oyarvide, Douglas A. Rubinson, Peter Kraft, Kimmie Ng, Ying Bao...** Vitamin D Levels Tied to Survival in Pancreatic Cancer. *Journal of clinical oncology.* [Online] June 2016. http://ascopubs.org/doi/abs/10.1200/JCO.2015.66.3005?sid=b7c6c7ae-2e2f-4dd4-a792-9a9bf7bc0884.

271. **Byers SW1, Rowlands T, Beildeck M, Bong YS.** Mechanism of action of vitamin D and the vitamin D receptor in colorectal cancer prevention and treatment. *PubMed.* [Online] Mar 2012. https://www.ncbi.nlm.nih.gov/pubmed/21861107.

272. Vitamin D & Colorectal Cancer. [Online] Mar 2015. http://www.hopkinscoloncancercenter.org/CMS/CMS_Page.aspx?CurrentUDV=59&CMS_Page_ID=AB041E4B-5568-46B9-8D12-BA3959A6F3F5.

273. **thompson, Dennis.** Vitamin D May Boost Colon Cancer Survival, Study Finds. *Health Day, News for Healthier Living.* [Online] Jan 12, 2015. https://consumer.healthday.com/cancer-information-5/colon-cancer-news-96/vitamin-d-may-boost-colon-cancer-survival-study-finds-695421.html.

274. **Yoon Ji Choi, Young Ha Kim, Chang Ho Cho, Sung Hi Kim, and Jung Eun Lee.** Circulating levels of vitamin D and colorectal adenoma: A case-control study and a meta-analysis. *PubMed.* [Online] Aug 7, 2015. https://www.ncbi.nlm.nih.gov/pmc/articles/PMC4528029/.

275. Inflammatory Bowel Disease. *Sutter Health Palo Alto Medical Foundation.* [Online] http://www.pamf.org/gastroenterology/conditions/inflammatory-bowel.html.

276. **Peterson, Riley.** Recent study finds that low vitamin D levels are associated with increased disease activity in ulcerative colitis. *Vitamin D Council.* [Online] Jul 14, 2016. https://www.vitamindcouncil.org/recent-study-finds-that-low-vitamin-d-levels-are-associated-with-increased-disease-activity-in-ulcerative-colitis/.

277. **Gubatan J1, Mitsuhashi S2, Zenlea T2, Rosenberg L2, Robson S2, Moss AC2.** Low vitamin D levels may increase the risk of ulcerative colitis relapse. *PubMed.* [Online] Feb 2017. https://www.ncbi.nlm.nih.gov/pubmed/27266980.

278. Hair Loss? It May Be Vitamin D Deficiency. *Progressive Health.* [Online] 2014. http://www.progressivehealth.com/hair-loss-vitamin-d.htm.

279. Martinez ME, Giovannucci EL, Colditz GA, et al. *Calcium, vitamin D, and the occurrence of colorectal cancer among women. J Natl Cancer Inst.* 88:1375-1382. 1996.

280. Salazar-Martinez E, Lazcano-Ponce EC, Gonzalez Lira-Lira G, Escudero-De los Rios P. *Nutritional determinants of epithelial ovarian cancer risk: a case-control study in Mexico. Oncology.* 63(2):151-7. 2002.

281. Thys-Jacobs S, Donovan D, Papadopoulos A, et al. *Vitamin D and calcium dysregulation in the polycystic ovarian syndrome. Steroids.* 64:430-435. 1999.

282. Cantorna M, Hayes C and DeLuca H. *1,25-Dihydroxycholecalciferol inhibits the progression of arthritis in murine models of human arthritis. Journal of Nutrition, v. 128, p. 68-72. 1998.*

283. Lemire J, Ince A and Takashima M. *1,25-dihydroxyvitamin D3 attenuates the expression of experimental murine lupus of MRL/l mice. Autoimmunity, v. 12, p. 143-148. 1992.*

284. Kearney J, Giovannucci E, Rimm EB, et al. *Calcium, vitamin D, and dairy foods and the occurrence of colon cancer in men. Am J Epidemiol.* 143:907-917. 1996.

285. **Ladegaard, Isak.** Cancer patients with high vitamin D levels live longer. *Science Nordic.* [Online] Aug 15, 2012. http://sciencenordic.com/cancer-patients-high-vitamin-d-levels-live-longer.

286. **Wagner, Carol L, Sarah N Taylor, Donna D Johnson, and Bruce W Hollis.** The role of vitamin D in pregnancy and lactation: emerging concepts. *PMC.* [Online] 2012. https://www.ncbi.nlm.nih.gov/pmc/articles/PMC4365424/.

287. **Lazebnik R, Eisenberg Z, Lazebnik N, Spirer Z, Weisman Y.** Vitamin D metabolites in amniotic fluid. *PubMed.* [Online] Mar 1983. https://www.ncbi.nlm.nih.gov/pubmed/6600461.

288. **counselling, Impact of maternal probiotic-supplemented dietary.** Impact of maternal probiotic-supplemented dietary counselling. *Cambridge.* [Online] 2010. https://www.cambridge.org/core/services/aop-cambridge-core/content/view/S0007114509993898.

289. Research suggests vitamin D supplementation reduces depression during pregnancy. *Vitamin D Council.* [Online] Sep 2016. https://www.vitamindcouncil.org/research-suggests-vitamin-d-supplementation-reduces-depression-during-pregnancy/.

290. Vitamin D helps reduce childhood allergy rate. *Medical Press.* [Online] Apr 2016. https://medicalxpress.com/news/2016-04-vitamin-d-childhood-allergy.html.

291. **Anne Merewood, Supriya D. Mehta, Tai C. Chen, Howard Bauchner, and Michael F. Holick.** Association between Vitamin D Deficiency and Primary Cesarean Section. *PubMed.* [Online] Mar 2009. https://www.ncbi.nlm.nih.gov/pmc/articles/PMC2681281/.

292. **Morales E, Guxens M, Llop S, Rodríguez-Bernal CL, Tardón A, Riaño I, Ibarluzea J, Lertxundi N, Espada M, Rodriguez A, Sunyer J; INMA Project.** Circulating 25-hydroxyvitamin D3 in pregnancy and infant neuropsychological development. *PubMed.* [Online] Oct 2012. https://www.ncbi.nlm.nih.gov/pubmed/22987876.

293. **function", Reprint of "Vitamin D deficiency in pregnant women impairs regulatory T cell.** Reprint of "Vitamin D deficiency in pregnant women impairs regulatory T cell function". [Online] Apr 2015. http://www.sciencedirect.com/science/article/pii/S0960076015000382.

294. **Etemadifar M1, Janghorbani M2.** Efficacy of high-dose vitamin D3 supplementation in vitamin D deficient pregnant women with multiple sclerosis: Preliminary findings of a randomized-controlled trial. *PubMed.* [Online] Apr 2015. https://www.ncbi.nlm.nih.gov/pubmed/26056550.

295. **Hanieh S1, Ha TT2, Simpson JA3, Thuy TT2, Khuong NC4, Thoang DD4, Tran TD5, Tuan T2, Fisher J6, Biggs BA7.** Maternal vitamin D status and infant outcomes in rural Vietnam: a prospective cohort study. *PubMed.* [Online] June 2014. https://www.ncbi.nlm.nih.gov/pubmed/24967813.

296. **Robert J. Schroth, Christopher Lavelle, Robert Tate, Sharon Bruce, Ronald J. Billings, Michael E.K. Moffatt.** Prenatal Vitamin D and Dental Caries in Infants. *AAP News and Journals.* [Online] Apr 2014. http://pediatrics.aappublications.org/content/early/2014/04/16/peds.2013-2215.

297. **Zhang C1, Qiu C, Hu FB, David RM, van Dam RM, Bralley A, Williams MA.** Maternal plasma 25-hydroxyvitamin D concentrations and the risk for gestational diabetes mellitus. *PubMed.* [Online] 2008. https://www.ncbi.nlm.nih.gov/pubmed/19015731.

298. **Boyles, Salynn.** High Doses of Vitamin D May Cut Pregnancy Risks. *WebMD.* [Online] 2010. www.webmd.com/baby/news/20100504/high-doses-of-vitamin-d-may-cut-pregnancy-risk#1.

299. **https://www.ncbi.nlm.nih.gov/pubmed/15734706.** The effects of iodine on intelligence in children: a meta-analysis of studies conducted in China. *PubMed.* [Online] https://www.ncbi.nlm.nih.gov/pubmed/15734706.

300. **Chang, Louise MD.** Vitamin D in Pregnancy May Be Key for Baby's Brain. *WebMD.* [Online] 2012. http://www.webmd.com/baby/news/20120920/vitamin-d-pregnancy-babys-brain#2.

301. Pregnancy and gestational vitamin D deficiency. *Vitamin D Council.* [Online] 2015. https://www.vitamindcouncil.org/newsletter-pregnancy-and-gestational-vitamin-d-deficiency/.

302. **Bodnar LM1, Krohn MA, Simhan HN.** Maternal vitamin D deficiency is associated with bacterial vaginosis in the first trimester of pregnancy. *PubMed.* [Online] Jun 2009. https://www.ncbi.nlm.nih.gov/pubmed/19357214.

303. **Merewood A1, Mehta SD, Chen TC, Bauchner H, Holick MF.** Association between vitamin D deficiency and primary cesarean section. *PubMed.* [Online] Mar 2009. https://www.ncbi.nlm.nih.gov/pubmed/19106272.

304. **Bodnar LM1, Catov JM, Simhan HN, Holick MF, Powers RW, Roberts JM.** Maternal vitamin D deficiency increases the risk of preeclampsia. *PubMed.* [Online] Sep 2007. https://www.ncbi.nlm.nih.gov/pubmed/17535985.

305. **Scholl TO1, Chen X.** Vitamin D intake during pregnancy: association with maternal characteristics and infant birth weight. *PubMed.* [Online] Apr 2009. https://www.ncbi.nlm.nih.gov/pubmed/19008055.

306. **Lee V1, Rekhi E, Hoh Kam J, Jeffery G.** Vitamin D rejuvenates aging eyes by reducing inflammation, clearing amyloid beta and improving visual function. *PubMed.* [Online] Oct 2012. https://www.ncbi.nlm.nih.gov/pubmed/22217419.

307. **Conin, Joseph.** Vitamin D Reportedly Improves Vision. *opticalceu.blogspot.* [Online] Jan 2012. http://opticalceu.blogspot.ch/2012/01/vitamin-d-reportedly-improves-vision.html.

308. **Bates, Claire.** Boosting vitamin D levels 'could help prevent eyesight from deteriorating'. *Mail Online.* [Online] Jan 2012. Boosting vitamin D levels 'could help prevent eyesight from deteriorating.

309. **Jenkins, Becca Borawski.** Vitamin D could help combat the effects of aging in eyes. *BIOTECHNOLOGY AND BIOLOGICAL SCIENCES RESEARCH COUNCIL.* [Online] JAN 2012. https://www.eurekalert.org/pub_releases/2012-01/babs-vdc011612.php.

310. **Lee V, Rekhi E, Hoh Kam J, Jeffery G.** Vitamin D rejuvenates aging eyes by reducing inflammation, clearing amyloid beta and improving visual function. *PubMed.* [Online] Oct 2012. https://www.ncbi.nlm.nih.gov/pubmed/22217419.

311. **Constantini NW1, Arieli R, Chodick G, Dubnov-Raz G.** High prevalence of vitamin D insufficiency in athletes and dancers. *PubMed.* [Online] Sep 2010. https://www.ncbi.nlm.nih.gov/pubmed/20818195.

312. **Fishman MP1, Lombardo SJ2, Kharrazi FD2.** Vitamin D Deficiency Among Professional Basketball Players. *PubMed.* [Online] Jul 2016. https://www.ncbi.nlm.nih.gov/pubmed/27482529.

313. **Cannell, John.** *Faster Quicker Stronger with vitamin D.* s.l. : Here & Now Books, 2011. ISBN: 978-0-9774272-9-1.

314. Cell Reports. *http://www.cell.com/cell-reports/abstract/S2211-1247(16)31362-6.* [Online] 10 26, 2016.

315. Vitamin D Engages Longevity Gene to Increase Lifespan: C. elegans Study. *Neuroscience News.* [Online] Oct 2016. http://neurosciencenews.com/vitamin-d-geneitcs-longevity-5354/.

316. **Mark, Karla PhD.** A new look at vitamin D challenges the current view of its benefits. *buckinstitute.* [Online] Oct 2016. http://www.buckinstitute.org/buck-news/new-look-vitamin-d-challenges-current-view-its-benefits.

317. **Holick, Michael PHD.** VITAMIN D: A D-LIGHTFUL SOLUTION FOR HEALTH. *PMC.* [Online] Aug 2011. https://www.ncbi.nlm.nih.gov/pmc/articles/PMC3738435/.

318. **Boucher, Barbara J.** The Problems of Vitamin D Insufficiency in Older People. *PMC.* [Online] Aug 2012. https://www.ncbi.nlm.nih.gov/pmc/articles/PMC3501367/.

319. **Annweiler C1, Schott AM, Allali G, Bridenbaugh SA, Kressig RW, Allain P, Herrmann FR, Beauchet O.** Association of vitamin D deficiency with cognitive impairment in older women: cross-sectional study. *PubMed.* [Online] Jan 2010. https://www.ncbi.nlm.nih.gov/pubmed/19794127.

320. **WE, Stumpf.** The endocrinology of sunlight and darkness. Complementary roles of vitamin D and pineal hormones. *PubMed.* [Online] May 1988. https://www.ncbi.nlm.nih.gov/pubmed/3043234.

321. **Editor .** Pineal Gland Calcification. *The Event Chronicle.* [Online] Dec 7, 2015. http://www.theeventchronicle.com/metaphysics/metascience/pineal-gland-calcification-why-you-should-care/#.

322. **Williams, Dr. David.** Your Pineal Gland Needs Protection. *Dr. David Williams.* [Online] http://www.drdavidwilliams.com/your-pineal-gland-needs-protection/.

323. **O'Connor, Clare, Ph.D.** Telomeres of Human Chromosomes. *Scitable .* [Online] 2008. http://art.daneshlink.ir/Handlera.ashx?server=1&id=21/scitable/topicpage/telomeres-of-human-chromosomes-21041.

324. **Tzanetako, IP, Nzietchueng R, Perrea DN, Benetos A1.** Telomeres and their role in aging and longevity. *PubMed.* [Online] 2014. https://www.ncbi.nlm.nih.gov/pubmed/24350925.

325. **Blackburn, Elizabeth MD, Elissa Eple PhD.** *The Telomere Effect: A Revolutionary Approach to Living Younger, Healthier, Longer.* s.l. : Grand Central Publishing, 2017. ISBN-13: 978-1455587971.

326. **Mohsen Mazidi, corresponding author1,2 Erin D. Michos,3,4 and Maciej Banach5,6.** The association of telomere length and serum 25-hydroxyvitamin D levels in US adults: the National Health and Nutrition Examination Survey. *PMC.* [Online] Feb 1, 2017. https://www.ncbi.nlm.nih.gov/pmc/articles/PMC5206371/.

327. **Richards, J Brent,Ana M Valdes, Jeffrey P Gardner, Dimitri Paximadas, Masayuki Kimura, Ayrun Nessa, Xiaobin Lu, Gabriela L Surdulescu, Rami Swaminathan, Tim D Spector, and Abraham Aviv.** Higher serum vitamin D concentrations are associated with longer leukocyte telomere length in women2. *PMC.* [Online] Jan 14, 2008. https://www.ncbi.nlm.nih.gov/pmc/articles/PMC2196219/.

328. **Rodrigo T. Calado, M.D., Ph.D.. and Bogdan Dumitriu, M.D.** Telomere dynamics in mice and humans. *PMC.* [Online] https://www.ncbi.nlm.nih.gov/pmc/articles/PMC3742037/.

329. **Tuohimaa, P.** Vitamin D and aging. *PubMed.* [Online] Mar 2009. https://www.ncbi.nlm.nih.gov/pubmed/?term=Tuohimaa%20P%5BAuthor%5D&cauthor=true&cauthor_uid=19444937.

330. **Haidong Zhu, MD PhD,1 Dehuang Guo, MD PhD,1 Ke Li, PhD,4 Jennifer Pedersen-White, DO,2 Inger Susanne Stallmann-Jorgensen, MS RD LD,1 Ying Huang, BS,1 Samip Parikh, MBBS MPH,1 Kebin Liu, PhD,3 and Yanbin Dong, MD PhD1.** Increased Telomerase Activity and Vitamin D Supplementation in Overweight African Americans. *PMC.* [Online] Nov 2013. https://www.ncbi.nlm.nih.gov/pmc/articles/PMC3826782/.

331. **Murnaghan, Ian BSc (hons), MS.** An Overview of DNA Functions. [Online] Jan 2017. http://www.exploredna.co.uk/an-overview-dna-functions.html.

332. **Harvey Lodish, Arnold Berk, S Lawrence Zipursky, Paul Matsudaira, David Baltimore, and James Darnell.** DNA Damage and Repair and Their Role in Carcinogenesis. [Online] 2000. https://www.ncbi.nlm.nih.gov/books/NBK21554/. ISBN-10: 0-7167-3136-3NCBI.

333. **Nair-Shalliker V, Armstrong BK, Fenech M.** Does vitamin D protect against DNA damage? *PubMed* . [Online] May 2012. https://www.ncbi.nlm.nih.gov/pubmed/22366026.

334. **Halicka HD1, Zhao H, Li J, Traganos F, Studzinski GP, Darzynkiewicz Z.** Attenuation of constitutive DNA damage signaling by 1,25-dihydroxyvitamin D3. *PubMed.* [Online] Apr 2012. https://www.ncbi.nlm.nih.gov/pubmed/22498490.

335. —. Attenuation of constitutive DNA damage signaling by 1,25-dihydroxyvitamin D3. *PubMed.* [Online] Apr 2012. https://www.ncbi.nlm.nih.gov/pubmed/22498490.

336. **James C. Fleet, 1,5 Marsha DeSmet,4 Robert Johnson,2 and Yan Li3.** Vitamin D and Cancer: A review of molecular mechanisms. *HHS Public Access.* [Online] Sep 2015. https://www.ncbi.nlm.nih.gov/pmc/about/public-access/.

337. History of Stem Cell Research. *Boston Children's Hospital.* [Online] http://stemcell.childrenshospital.org/about-stem-cells/history/.

338. HISTORY OF STEM CELL RESEARCH — A TIMELINE. *About Stem Cells.* [Online] http://stemcell.childrenshospital.org/about-stem-cells/history/.

339. **Maximow, alexander A.** The lymphocyte as a stem cell, common to different blood elements in embryonic development and during the post-fetal life of mammals. *Cellular Therapy and Transplantation.* [Online] June 1909. http://www.ctt-journal.com/1-3-en-maximow-1909-translation.html.

340. E. Donnall Thomas, M.D. *Stem Cells Translational Medicine.* [Online] https://www.ncbi.nlm.nih.gov/pmc/articles/PMC3659750/.

341. **Gluckman E, Rocha V.** History of the clinical use of umbilical cord blood hematopoietic cells. *PubMed.* [Online] 2005. https://www.ncbi.nlm.nih.gov/pubmed/16081348.

342. What are stem cells? How are they regulated? *U.S. Food & Drug Administration.* [Online] https://www.fda.gov/AboutFDA/Transparency/Basics/ucm194655.htm.

343. **Murnaghan, Ian BSc (hons), MSc.** History of Stem Cell Research. *Explore Stem cells* . [Online] Feb 3, 2017. http://www.explorestemcells.co.uk/historystemcellresearch.html.

344. **Harris, David T University of Arizona, Department of Immunobiology, e.al.** The potential of cord blood stem cells for use in regenerative medicine. *Taylor Francis Online.* [Online] Aug 2007. http://www.tandfonline.com/doi/abs/10.1517/14712598.7.9.1311?journalCode=iebt20&.

345. 1358 studies found for cord blood . *Clinical Trials.Gov.* [Online] https://clinicaltrials.gov/ct2/results?term=cord+blood&Search=Search.

346. Blu Room . [Online] 2017. http://www.bluroom.com/emailers/0123_NWS/online_STY.html.

347. The Medical Promise of Stem Cells. *Regenerative Medicine Stem Cell Therapy.* [Online] http://stemcellpromise.yolasite.com/stem-cell.php.

348. **Trounson A1, McDonald C2.** Clinical trials for stem cell therapies. *PubMed.* [Online] Jul 2, 2015. https://www.ncbi.nlm.nih.gov/pubmed/26140604.

349. **Hall, Aric C. and Mark B. Juckett.** The Role of Vitamin D in Hematologic Disease and Stem Cell Transplantation. *PMC.* [Online] Jun 2013. https://www.ncbi.nlm.nih.gov/pmc/articles/PMC3725501/.

350. **Smith, Robin L,M.D. Tomasz Trafny, Max Gomez Ph.D.** *the Healing Cell.* New York : Center Street, Hachette Book Group, 2013. ISBN: 978-1-4555-7292-2.

351. **Harris Dt., Rogers.** Umbilical cord blood: a unique source of pluripotent stem cells for regenerative medicine. *PubMed.* [Online] Dec 2007. https://www.ncbi.nlm.nih.gov/pubmed/18220914.

352. What is the difference between totipotent, pluripotent, and multipotent? [Online] https://stemcell.ny.gov/faqs/what-difference-between-totipotent-pluripotent-and-multipotent .

353. Stem Cell Information. *National Institues of Health.* [Online] https://stemcells.nih.gov/info/basics/4.htm.

354. **Siegel, Georg, Torsten Kluba, Ursula Hermanutz-Klein, Karen Bieback,3 Hinnak Northoff,1 and Richard Schäfercorresponding author1,4.** Phenotype, donor age and gender affect function of human bone marrow-derived mesenchymal stromal cells. *PMC.* [Online] Jun 11, 2013. https://www.ncbi.nlm.nih.gov/pmc/articles/PMC3694028/.

355. **Munoz J1, Shah N2, Rezvani K1, Hosing C1, Bollard CM1, Oran B1, Olson A1, Popat U1, Molldrem J1, McNiece IK1, Shpall EJ1.** Concise review: umbilical cord blood transplantation: past, present, and future. *PubMed.* [Online] Dec 2014. https://www.ncbi.nlm.nih.gov/pubmed/25378655.

356. **Weiss, Mark L., Troyer Deryl.** Stem Cells in the Umbilical Cord. *PMC.* [Online] Aug 26, 2013. https://www.ncbi.nlm.nih.gov/pmc/articles/PMC3753204/.

357. **Hiyama, E and K Hiyama.** Telomere and telomerase in stem cells. *PMC.* [Online] pr 2007. https://www.ncbi.nlm.nih.gov/pmc/articles/PMC2360127/.

358. **Kasiappan, Ravi, Zheng Shen,Anfernee K-W Tse, Umesh Jinwal, Jinfu Tang,Panida Lungchukiet,Yuefeng Sun,Patricia Kruk, Santo V. Nicosia, Xiaohong Zhang, and Wenlong Bai.** 1,25-Dihydroxyvitamin D3 Suppresses Telomerase Expression and Human Cancer Growth through MicroRNA-498. *PMC.* [Online] Nov 2012. https://www.ncbi.nlm.nih.gov/pmc/articles/PMC3510828/.

359. **Hal,Aric C.* and Mark B. Juckett.** The Role of Vitamin D in Hematologic Disease and Stem Cell Transplantation. *PMC.* [Online] Jun 2013. https://www.ncbi.nlm.nih.gov/pmc/articles/PMC3725501/.

360. http://www.sciencedirect.com/science/article/pii/S1083879114003309#. Vitamin D Levels Affect Outcome in Pediatric Hematopoietic Stem Cell Transplantation. [Online] Oct 2014. http://www.sciencedirect.com/science/article/pii/S1083879114003309.

361. **Gu SG1, Wang CJ, Zhao G, Li GY.** Role of vitamin D in regulating the neural stem cells of mouse model with multiple sclerosis. *PubMed.* [Online] Nov 2015. https://www.ncbi.nlm.nih.gov/pubmed/26592821.

362. Vitamin D increases the number of blood stem cells during embryonic development. [Online] Oct 4, 2016. https://www.eurekalert.org/pub_releases/2016-10/cp-vdi100316.php.

363. **Posa, Francesca,1 Adriana Di Benedetto,1 Graziana Colaianni,2 Elisabetta A. Cavalcanti-Adam,3,4 Giacomina Brunetti,2 Chiara Porro,1 Teresa Trotta,1 Maria Grano,2 and Giorgio Mori1.** Vitamin D Effects on Osteoblastic Differentiation of Mesenchymal Stem Cells from Dental Tissues. *Stem Cells International.* [Online] 2016. https://www.hindawi.com/journals/sci/2016/9150819/.

364. **Haussler MR, Haussler CA, Whitfield GK, Hsieh JC, Thompson PD, Barthel TK, Bartik L, Egan JB, Wu Y, Kubicek JL, Lowmiller CL, Moffet EW, Forster RE, Jurutka PW.** The nuclear vitamin D receptor controls the expression of genes encoding factors which feed the "Fountain of Youth" to mediate healthful aging. *PubMed.* [Online] Mar 20, 2010. https://www.ncbi.nlm.nih.gov/pubmed/20227497.

365. **Jonny Bowden.** Vitamin D: The "Real" Fountain Of Youth? *JB Jonny Bowden.* [Online] May 4, 2010. https://www.jonnybowden.com/vitamin-d-fountain-of-youth/.

366. Ultraviolettstrahlung. *Welt der Physik.* [Online] March 2006. http://www.weltderphysik.de/gebiet/atome/elektromagnetisches-spektrum/ultraviolettstrahlung/.

367. **Darielle.** History of Ultraviolet Ligh. *Good Changes Now.* [Online] Apr 2013. http://goodchangesnowblog.com/history-of-ultraviolet-light/.

368. ST. PETERSBURG UPGRADES WATER TREATMENT PLANTS WITH UV SYSTEMS. [Online] http://www.waterworld.com/articles/wwi/print/volume-20/issue-10/features/st-petersburg-upgrades-water-treatment-plants-with-uv-systems.html.

369. UV Lights to Sanitize a St. Petersburg Air Conditioner. [Online] 2006. https://de.scribd.com/document/233875106/UV-Lights-to-Sanitize-a-St-Petersburg-Air-Conditioner.

370. Sterilizable washing machine using ultraviolet radiation and sterilizable washing method in the same. *Patentresearch.* [Online] 2009. http://www.google.ch/patents/US8303718?utm_source=gb-gplus-sharePatent.

371. Ultravoilet, antibacterial, antifungal dryerlight . *Patents.* [Online] Sep 9, 1997. https://www.google.com/patents/US5664340.

372. LG's latest TrueSteam dishwasher can disinfect your crockery with an integrated UV lamp, which should kill up to 99% of bacteria. *expert reviews.* [Online] March 19, 2014. http://www.expertreviews.co.uk/accessories/gadgets/27808/lg-truesteam-dishwasher-blasts-bugs-with-uv-lamp.

373. Helix 450XL Total Toom UV Sanitizer. [Online] http://www.mrsa-uv.com/products.html.

374. **Helman, Christopher.** How A New Machine Uses U.V. Rays To Blast Killer Bacteria. [Online] Nov 2, 2011. https://www.forbes.com/sites/christopherhelman/2011/11/02/bug-zapper-how-a-new-machine-snuffs-killer-bacteria-with-ultraviolet-blasts/#1cde4b1c237c.

375. **Helman, Christopher.** http://www.forbes.com/sites/christopherhelman/2011/11/02/bug-zapper-how-a-new-machine-snuffs-killer-bacteria-with-ultraviolet-blasts. *Forbes.* [Online] Nov 2, 2011. http://www.forbes.com/sites/christopherhelman/2011/11/02/bug-zapper-how-a-new-machine-snuffs-killer-bacteria-with-ultraviolet-blasts/#428865c411a7.

376. Photoluminescence Therapy Curing Many Illnesses. [Online] 2014. http://undergroundhealthreporter.com/photoluminescence-therapy/.

377. **Rowen, Robert Jay.** The Cure that Time forgot - Ultraviolet Blood Irradiation Therapy (Photo-Oxidation). *Foundation For Biosocial Research.* [Online] 1996. http://www.vitamind.arcarmichael.com/Irradiation/rowen.htm.

378. **Havasi, Peter.** *Education of Cancer Healing Vol. VII-Heretics.* s.l. : Lulu, 2012. ISBN: 978-1-291-45368-3.

379. UV Light Part III Photoluminescence Therapy. [Online] 2006. http://www.mnwelldir.org/docs/uv_light/uv_light3.htm.

380. Ultraviolet Blood Therapy (Photoluminescence). *Drummartin Clinic.* [Online] 1996. http://www.integrativemedonline.com/illness_blood_theraphy.html.

381. **Havasi, Peter.** *Education of Cancer Healing Vol. VII -.* s.l. : Lulu.com, 1994. ISBN: 1291453687, 9781291453683.

382. **Gilchrest BA, Rowe JW, Brown RS, Steinman TI, Arndt KA.** Relief of uremic pruritus with ultraviolet phototherapy. *PubMed.* [Online] Jul 1977. https://www.ncbi.nlm.nih.gov/pubmed/865585/.

383. **Kuenstner JT, Mukherjee S, Weg S, Landry T, Petrie T.** The treatment of infectious disease with a medical device: results of a clinical trial of ultraviolet blood irradiation (UVBI) in patients with hepatitis C infection. *PubMed.* [Online] Aug 2015. https://www.ncbi.nlm.nih.gov/pubmed/26092299.

384. **Shirazian, Shayan, Olufemi Aina, Youngjun Park, Nawsheen Chowdhury,1 Kathleen Leger, Linle Hou, Nobuyuki Miyawaki, and Vandana S Mathur.** Chronic kidney disease-associated pruritus: impact on quality of life and current management challenges. *PMC.* [Online] Jan 2017. https://www.ncbi.nlm.nih.gov/pmc/articles/PMC5271405/.

385. Blu Room. [Online] http://www.bluroom.com/.

386. **Bertone, Nikki.** Nikki Bertones Story. [Online] Jan 2017. http://bluroom.com/emailers/0123_NWS/online_STY.html.

387. **Reimann, Costas A. Anastassiou, Rodrigo Perin, Sean L. Hill, Henry Markram, Christof Koch.** A Biophysically Detailed Model of Neocortical Local Field Potentials Predicts the Critical Role of Active Membrane Currents. [Online] July 2013. https://www.sciencedaily.com/releases/2013/07/130724124911.htm.

388. What are Brainwaves. *brainworks.* [Online] http://www.brainworksneurotherapy.com/what-are-brainwaves.

389. Learn about the Wonders of Theta Medidation Music. *Binaural Beats Medidation.* [Online] https://www.binauralbeatsmeditation.com/the-wonders-of-theta-meditation-music/.

390. **Herrmann, Ned.** What is the function of the various brainwaves? [Online] 1997. https://www.scientificamerican.com/article/what-is-the-function-of-t-1997-12-22/.

391. **Ehlers, Cindy, David Kupfer.** Slow-wave sleep: do young adult men and women age differently? *Wiley Online Library.* [Online] Sep 1997. http://onlinelibrary.wiley.com/doi/10.1046/j.1365-2869.1997.00041.x/abstract;jsessionid=2F8D29EE14262535F748E16FC5FA4BB1.f03t04.

392. **Bergland, Christopher.** Alpha Brain Waves Boost Creativity and Reduce Depression. *Psychology Today.* [Online] Apr 2015. https://www.psychologytoday.com/blog/the-athletes-way/201504/alpha-brain-waves-boost-creativity-and-reduce-depression.

393. The Benefits of Gamma Brainwaves. *Brainwave Wizard.* [Online] http://brainwavewizard.com/entrainment/the-benefits-of-gamma-brainwaves/.

394. What are Brainwaves. [Online] http://www.brainworksneurotherapy.com/what-are-brainwaves.

395. **Heather, Simon.** Om – The Primordial Sound by Simon Heather. [Online] http://www.simonheather.co.uk/pages/articles/aum.pdf.

396. Schumann Resonance. *Blisscoded Sound.* [Online] http://blisscodedsound.com/schumann-resonance/.

397. The Secret Behind 432 Hz Tuning. *The Bell Tower Project.* [Online] http://belltowerproject.com/the-secret-behind-432hz-tuning/.

398. The secret behind 432 Hz tuning. [Online] 2016. https://attunedvibrations.com/432hz-healing/.

399. 432 Hz – Unearthing the Truth Behind Nature's Frequency. *Binaural Beats medidation.* [Online] https://www.binauralbeatsmeditation.com/432-hz-truth-behind-natures-frequency/.

400. A440 pitch standard. [Online] https://en.wikipedia.org/wiki/A440_(pitch_standard).

401. **St-Onge, Elina.** HERE'S WHY YOU SHOULD CONSIDER CONVERTING YOUR MUSIC TO A=432 HZ. *CE Collective Evolution.* [Online] Dec 21, 2013. http://www.collective-evolution.com/2013/12/21/heres-why-you-should-convert-your-music-to-432hz/.

402. **Foster, Brian.** Einstein's Universe. [Online] 2001. http://www.einsteinsuniverse.com/Einsteins_Universe/Einsteins_Universe.html.

403. **Miller, Arthur I.** A Genius Finds Inspiration in the Music of Another. *New York Times.* [Online] Jan31 2006. http://www.nytimes.com/2006/01/31/science/a-genius-finds-inspiration-in-the-music-of-another.html.

404. What are the Solfeggio frequencies? *Attuned vibrations.* [Online] 1996. https://attunedvibrations.com/solfeggio/.

405. The Sacred Solfeggio Frequencies. [Online] http://www.warrior-priestess.com/12strandDNA-Solfeggio.html.

406. Water. [Online] 2005. http://www.whatthebleep.com/water-crystals/.

407. Forgotten In Time: The Ancient Solfeggio Frequencies. *RED ICE CREATION.* [Online] 2006. http://www.redicecreations.com/specialreports/2006/01jan/solfeggio.html.

408. **Gottschalk,Kirsten under the supervision of Paul Francis.** Sounds of the Universe. *Sounds of the Universe.* [Online] 2004. http://www.mso.anu.edu.au/pfrancis/Music/index.html.

409. NASA Spacecraft Records 'Earthsong. *NASA Science Beta.* [Online] Oct 1, 2012. https://www.nasa.gov/mp3/687631main_687014main_emfisis_chorus_1.mp3.

410. The origin of time and the secret of nine. *Trace Elements Radio.* [Online] 2015. http://www.traceelementsradio.com/2015/12/the-origin-of-time-and-secret-of-nine.html.

411. Egypt unlocked. [Online] http://www.egyptunlocked.com/blog/the-origin-of-time-and-the-secret-of-nine/.

412. Significance of Number Nine in Vedas. [Online] 2010. http://mathomathis.blogspot.ch/2010/08/vedas-mathematics.html.

413. **Guthrie, Kenneth Sylvan.** *The Pythagorean Sourcebook and Library.* s.l. : Phanes Press, 1987. ISBN 0-933999-51-8.

414. **Finton Ken.** The Geometry of Circles. [Online] Jul 2015. https://kennethfinton.com/2015/07/26/the-geometry-of-circles/.

415. **Venefica, Avia.** Symbolic meaning of Octagon. *symbolic meanings.* [Online] May 2008. http://www.symbolic-meanings.com/2008/05/24/symbolic-meaning-of-octagon/.

416. Tesla Tower in Shoreham Long Island (1901 - 1917) meant to be the "World Wireless" Broadcasting system. *Tesla memorial Society of New York.* [Online] http://www.teslasociety.com/teslatower.htm.

417. **(Alhazen), A-Haytham.** *The Optics of Ibn Al-Haytham: On Direct Vision Books .* s.l. : Warburg Institute; First Edition edition (December 1, 1989), 1989. ISBN-13: 978-0854810727.

418. Introduction top the Reflection of Light. *Microscopy Resource Center.* [Online] 2006. http://www.olympusmicro.com/primer/lightandcolor/reflectionintro.html.

419. Introduction to the Reflection of Light. *Microscopy Resource Center.* [Online] 2006. http://www.olympusmicro.com/primer/lightandcolor/reflectionintro.html.

420. The Law of Vibration. *One Mind - One energy.* [Online] http://www.one-mind-one-energy.com/Law-of-vibration.html.

421. The Law of Vibration. [Online] http://www.natural-health-zone.com/law-of-vibration.html.

422. Frequency & the Law of Vibration. [Online] Jul 18, 2010. https://hiddenlighthouse.wordpress.com/2010/07/18/frequency-the-law-of-vibration/.

423. Tesla coil. [Online] https://en.wikipedia.org/wiki/Tesla_coil.

424. **Brown Tom.** Tesla Coil - Lost Inventions of Nikola Tesla. [Online] http://altered-states.net/barry/newsletter208/.

425. **Sills, Franklin.** *The Breath of Life, Holism and Biodynamics.* Berkeley CA : North Atlantic Books, 2011.

426. Viktor Schauberger. [Online] http://schauberger.co.uk/.

427. **Fraser, Peter, Harry Massey r.** *Decoding the Human Body-Field: The New Science of Information as Medicine,.* s.l. : Healings Arts Press , 2008.

428. **Chiganças V1, Miyaji EN, Muotri AR, de Fátima Jacysyn J, Amarante-Mendes GP, Yasui A, Menck CF.** Photorepair prevents ultraviolet-induced apoptosis in human cells expressing the marsupial photolyase gene. *PubMed.* [Online] May 2000. https://www.ncbi.nlm.nih.gov/pubmed/10811124.

429. **Eden, Dan .** Dr. Fritz-Albert Popp thought he had discovered a cure for cancer. *Bioontology ARIZONA.* [Online] http://www.biontologyarizona.com/fritz-albert-popp-cure-for-cancer/.

430. **Popp, Prof. Dr. F.A.** *Biophotonen- Neue Horizonte in der Medizin. Von den Grundlagen zur Biophoton 2006.* 2006. ISBN-10: 3830472676.

431. **Ji, Sayer.** Biophotons: The Human Body is Made from Coherent Light. *The Event Chronicle.* [Online] March 2017. http://www.theeventchronicle.com/metaphysics/metascience/biophotons-human-body-made-coherent-light/.

432. **Kruse, Jack.** Quantum Biology 1: The Zero Entropy System. *Reversing disease for optimal health.* [Online] 2013. https://www.jackkruse.com/quantum-biology-1-the-zero-entropy-system/.

433. Stuart R. Hameroff, MD. *Arizona Health Science s Center.* [Online] 2016. http://anesth.medicine.arizona.edu/faculty/stuart-r-hameroff-md.

434. Prof. Sir R. Penrose. *Mathematical Physics.* [Online] https://www.maths.ox.ac.uk/people/roger.penrose.

435. Discovery of Quantum Vibrations in "Microtubules" Inside Brain Neurons Corroborates Controversial 20-Year-Old Theory of Consciousness. [Online] Jan 2014. https://www.elsevier.com/about/press-releases/research-and-journals/discovery-of-quantum-vibrations-in-microtubules-inside-brain-neurons-corroborates-controversial-20-year-old-theory-of-consciousness.

436. **Bortfeldt, Kerstin M.D.** Das Wunder in den Mikrotubuli . *Instatera Blu Room Weimar.* [Online] Mar 14, 2016. http://instatera.de/das-wunder-in-den-mikrotubuli-ii/.

437. **vitamin, Vitamin D: The "sunshine".** Vitamin D: The "sunshine" vitamin. *PMC.* [Online] Apr 2012. https://www.ncbi.nlm.nih.gov/pmc/articles/PMC3356951/.

438. **Barbarosa-Canovas, Gustavo V.** *Water Activity in Foods: Fundamentals and Applications.* s.l. : Blackwell Publishing, 2007.

439. Dr. Gerald Pollack, and Structured Water Science. *Structured Water Articles.* [Online] 2011. https://www.structuredwaterunit.com/articles/structuredwater/dr-gerald-pollack-and-structured-water-science.

440. **Jobs, Steve.** Steve Jobs – die Kreativität und sein kohärentes Feld. *Zeit und Raum.* [Online] Oct 10, 2011. http://zeitundraum.blogspot.ch/2011/10/steve-jobs-die-kreativitat-und-sein.html.

441. A collection of audiovisual stimulation study abstracts from the beginning to the present. *neurotronics.* [Online] 2010. http://www.neurotronics.eu/index.php?id=studien-details&L=2&ref=social&cmp=Test&tx_ttnews%5Btt_news%5D=31&tx_ttnews%5Bpointer%5D=1&cHash=06a4e210b2d27dedaaddc54ee5daaa3d.

442. Theta Brain Waves. *BINAURAL beats geek.* [Online] 2012. http://www.binauralbeatsgeek.com/theta-brain-waves/.

443. **Birbaumer, Niels, PhD, PhD hc.** Tom Budzynski, The Hero of Neurofeedback. [Online] 2011. http://www.aapb-biofeedback.com/doi/abs/10.5298/1081-5937-39.4.04?code=aapb-site&journalCode=biof.

444. **Harris DT1, Rogers I.** Umbilical cord blood: a unique source of pluripotent stem cells for regenerative medicine. *PubMed.* [Online] Dec 2007. https://www.ncbi.nlm.nih.gov/pubmed/18220914.

445. What is Cord Blood? [Online] https://www.cordblood.com/benefits-cord-blood.

446. **Just, William, Ignacio Floresa, Maria A. Blascob, .** The role of telomeres and telomerase in stem cell aging. [Online] 2010. http://www.sciencedirect.com/science/article/pii/S0014579310006046.

447. Stem Cells for the Treatment of Type 1 Diabetes. *CryoCell.* [Online] https://www.cryo-cell.com/diabetes/stem-cells-for-the-treatment-of-type-i-diabetes.

448. **Alireza Rezania, Jennifer E Bruin, Payal Arora, Allison Rubin, Irina Batushansky, Ali Asadi, Shannon O'Dwyer, Nina Quiskamp, Majid Mojibian, Tobias Albrecht, Yu Hsuan Carol Yang, James D Johnson & Timothy J Kieffer.** Reversal of diabetes with insulin-producing cells derived in vitro from human pluripotent stem cells. *Nature Biotechnology 32, 1121–1133 (2014) doi:10.1038/nbt.3033.* [Online] Sep 2014. http://www.nature.com/nbt/journal/v32/n11/full/nbt.3033.html.

449. **Jaspen, Bruce.** Heart Therapy with Stem Cells Shows Progress. *CrycoCell.* [Online] https://www.cryo-cell.com/heart-disease/heart-therapy-with-stem-cells-shows-progress.

450. How are cord blood stem cells sving lives now? *CrycoCell.* [Online] https://www.cryo-cell.com/cord-blood-treating-diseases.

451. First paralyzed human treated with stem cells has now regained his upper body movement. [Online] http://theheartysoul.com/stem-cells-cure-paralysis/.

452. **Fox, Michael.** Stem Cells and Parkinson's Disease. *the Michael J. Fox Foundation.* [Online] 2012. https://www.michaeljfox.org/understanding-parkinsons/living-with-pd/topic.php?stem-cells.

453. **Martinez, Dr. Matthew.** *Der BLU ROOM™ und dessen Wirkung auf Körper und Geist von Dr. Matthew Martinez.* Klagenfurt Austria : BluRelax Kalgenfurt, 2017. https://www.youtube.com/watch?v=ZaqfiY_4GWw.

454. **Gräf, Irmgard Maria.** *Mein Blut - ein Weg zu mir.* Peiting : Michaels Verlag, 2014.

455. **Menning, Hans.** *Das psychische Immunsystem.* Göttingen : Hogrefe Verlag, 2015. ISBN 978-3-8017-2495-5.

456. *Blut - Highway des Lebens.* **Gräf.** s.l. : Matrix3000, Vol. 86.

457. pubmed. *https://www.ncbi.nlm.nih.gov/pubmed/24494042.* [Online] 2013.

458. pubmed. *https://www.ncbi.nlm.nih.gov/pmc/articles/PMC3897598/.* [Online] 2013.

459. **Hess, A.** The history of rickets. In:Rickets, Including Osteomalacia and Tetany Lea & Febiger. *Hess A. The history of rickets. In:Rickets, Including Osteomalacia and Tetany Lea & Febiger: Philadelphia, 1929; pp22–37.* Philadelphia : s.n., 1929; pp22–37.

460. **JM., Mitric.** *Mitric JM. Maturity News Service, November 15, 1992.* Maturity News Service : s.n., 1992.

461. **RR., Recker.** *Recker RR. Osteoporosis. Contemporary Nutrition, Vol. 8, no. 5, May 1983.* s.l. : Contemporary Nutrition, 1983.

462. **SW, Key.** *Key SW, Marble M. Studies link sun exposure to protection against cancer. Cancer Weekly Plus. November 17, 1997: 5-6.* Cancer Weekly Plus. November 17, 1997 : s.n., 1997.

463. **Studzinski GP, Moore DC.** *Studzinski GP, Moore DC. Sunlight: can it prevent as well as cause cancer? Cancer Res. 55:4014-4022. 1995.* Cancer Res. 55:4014-4022. 1995 : s.n., 1995.

464. **F, Cosman.** *Cosman F, Nieves J, Komar L, Ferrer G, Herbert J, Formica C, Shen V, Lindsay R. Fracture history and bone loss in patients with MS. Neurology. Oct; 51(4):1161-5. 1998.* Neurology. Oct; 51(4):1161-5. 1998 : s.n., 1998.

465. **CE, Hayes.** *Hayes CE, Cantorna MT, DeLuca HF. Vitamin D and multiple sclerosis. Proc Soc Exp Biol Med. Oct; 216(1):21-27. 1997.* Proc Soc Exp Biol Med. Oct; 216(1):21-27. 1997 : 1997.

466. **R, Scragg.** *Scragg R. Sunlight, vitamin D, and cardiovascular disease. In: Crass MF II, Avioli LV, eds. Calcium Regulating Hormones and Cardiovascular Function. Boca Raton, Fla: CRC Press; 213-237. 1995.* CRC Press; 213-237. 1995 : s.n., 1995.

467. **MR, Werbach.** *Werbach MR and Moss J. Textbook of Nutritional Medicine. Tarzana, Calif: Third Line Press; 1999. p 423.* Third Line Press; 1999. p 423 : s.n., 1999.

468. Bicknell F and Prescott F. *The Vitamins in Medicine, third edition. Milwaukee, WI: Lee Foundation. p 573. 1953.*

469. Cantorna MT, Munsick C, Bemiss C, Mahon BD. *1,25-Dihydroxycholecalciferol prevents and ameliorates symptoms of experimental murine inflammatory bowel disease. J Nutr. Nov; 130(11):2648-52. 2000.*

470. Yeste D and Carrascosa A. *[Nutritional rickets in childhood: analysis of 62 cases][Article in Spanish] Med Clin (Barc). Jun 7;121(1):23-7. 2003.*

471. Goldberg P. *Multiple Sclerosis: vitamin D and calcium as environmental determinants of prevalence. Part 1: Sunlight, dietary factors and epidemiology. Intern. J. Environmental Studies, v. 6, p. 19-27. 1974.*

472. **Veugelers, Paul J. and John Paul Ekwaru.** *A Statistical Error in the Estimation of the Recommended.* Nutrients 2014, 6, 4472-4475; doi:10.3390/nu6104472 : s.n.

473. Embry AF. *Vitamin D supplementation in the fight against multiple sclerosis. http://www.direct-ms.org/vitamind.html Accessed July, 2003.*

474. https://www.ncbi.nlm.nih.gov/pmc/articles/PMC3897598/. *Caldwell M, Flint S. Stratospheric ozone reduction, solar UV-B radiation and terrestrial ecosystems. Clim Change. 1994;28:375–94. doi: 10.1007/BF01104080.* [Online]

475. Rostand SG. *Ultraviolet light may contribute to geographic and racial blood pressure differences. Hypertension. 1997;30:150–6. doi: 10.1161/01.HYP.30.2.150.* https://www.ncbi.nlm.nih.gov/pmc/articles/PMC3897598/ : s.n.

476. Huldschinsky K. *The ultra-violet light treatment of rickets. Alpine Press New Jersey, USA 1928;3–19.* https://www.ncbi.nlm.nih.gov/pmc/articles/PMC3897598/ : s.n.

477. the bmj Research. *http://www.bmj.com/content/348/bmj.g3656.* [Online] 6 17, 2014.

478. US National Library of Medicine. *https://www.ncbi.nlm.nih.gov/pmc/articles/PMC4806418/.* [Online] 3 2016.

479. **Brewer, L.C., Michos, E.D. & Reis, J.P.** *Vitamin D in atherosclerosis.* Current Drug Targets 12 54-60 : s.n., 2011.

480. **Husain, K., Ferder, L., Mizobuchi, M. et al.** *Combination therapy with paricalcitol and enalapril ameliorates cardiac oxidative injury in uremic rats.* American Journal of Nephrology, 29, 465 : s.n., 2009.

481. VitaminDWiki. *http://www.vitamindwiki.com/Allergy+-+Overview#Food_Allergy_5X_more_likely_if_low_vitamin_D_Oct_2014.* [Online] Oct 2014.

482. **Sidbury R, Sullivan AF, Thadhani RI, Camargo CA., Jr.** https://www.ncbi.nlm.nih.gov/pmc/articles/PMC2914320/. *Randomized controlled trial of vitamin D supplementation for winter-related atopic dermatitis in Boston: a pilot study. Br J Dermatol. .* [Online] 2008.

483. **Feuille, Elizabeth J., Anna H. Nowak-Węgrzyn.** Vitamin D Insufficiency Is Associated With Challenge-Proven Food Allergy in Infants. *http://pediatrics.aappublications.org/content/132/Supplement_1/S7.short#.* [Online] Oct 2013.

484. **Spedding, Simon.** Vitamin D and Depression: A Systematic Review and Meta-Analysis Comparing Studies with and without Biological Flaws. *NCBI.* [Online] Apr 2014. https://www.ncbi.nlm.nih.gov/pmc/articles/PMC4011048/.

485. **Gouni-Berthold I1, Krone W, Berthold HK.** Vitamin D and cardiovascular disease. *PubMed.* [Online] Jul 2009. https://www.ncbi.nlm.nih.gov/pubmed/19601865.

486. **Stefan Pilz, Andreas Tomaschitz, Winfried Maerz–, Christiane Drechsler, Eberhard Ritz‡‡, Armin Zittermann‡‡, Etienne Cavalier Thomas R. Pieber, Joan M. Lappe, William B. Grant, Michael F. Holick and Jacqueline M. Dekker.** Vitamin D, cardiovascular disease and mortality. *Wiley Online Library.* [Online] Oct 4, 2011. http://onlinelibrary.wiley.com/doi/10.1111/j.1365-2265.2011.04147.x/full.

487. **Pilz, S., Iodice, S., Zittermann, A. et al.** Vitamin D status and mortality risk in chronic kidney disease: a meta-analysis of prospective studies. *PubMed.* [Online] Sep 2011. https://www.ncbi.nlm.nih.gov/pubmed/21636193.

488. **Stefan Pilz, Andreas Tomaschitz, Winfried Maerz–, Christiane Drechsler, Eberhard Ritz††, Armin Zittermann#‡, Etienne Cavalier Thomas R. Pieber, Joan M. Lappe, William B. Grant, Michael F. Holick and Jacqueline M. Dekker.** *Vitamin D, cardiovascular disease and mortality.* Clinical Endocrinology : s.n., 2011.

489. **Lehmann B1, Rudolph T, Pietzsch J, Meurer M.** Conversion of vitamin D3 to 1alpha,25-dihydroxyvitamin D3 in human skin equivalents. *NCBI.* [Online] Apr 9, 2000. https://www.ncbi.nlm.nih.gov/pubmed/10772383.

490. **Rodríguez M, Daniels B, Gunawardene S, Robbins GK.** High frequency of vitamin D deficiency in ambulatory HIV-Positive patients. *PubMed.* [Online] Jan 25, 2009. https://www.ncbi.nlm.nih.gov/pubmed/19108690.

491. **Cannell JJ1, Vieth R, Umhau JC, Holick MF, Grant WB, Madronich S, Garland CF, Giovannucci E.** Epidemic influenza and vitamin D. *PubMed.* [Online] Dec 2006. https://www.ncbi.nlm.nih.gov/pubmed/16959053.

492. **Gotzsche, PC.** Niels Finsen's treatment for lupus vulgaris. *PMC.* [Online] Jan 1, 2011. https://www.ncbi.nlm.nih.gov/pmc/articles/PMC3014565/.

493. **Swanson,Jerry W. M.D.** Is there any proof that vitamin D supplements can prevent MS or keep symptoms of MS from worsening? *Mayo Clinic.* [Online] Feb 04, 2016. http://www.mayoclinic.org/diseases-conditions/multiple-sclerosis/expert-answers/vitamin-d-and-ms/faq-20058258.

494. **Wedad Z. Mostafa, , Rehab A. Hegazy.** Vitamin D and the skin: Focus on a complex relationship: A review. *ScienceDirect.* [Online] 2014. http://www.sciencedirect.com/science/article/pii/S209012321400023X.

495. **Bikle, Daniel D.** Vitamin D metabolism and function in the skin. [Online] Dec 5, 2011. http://www.sciencedirect.com/science/article/pii/S0303720711002590.

496. **Alberts B, Johnson A, Lewis J, et al.** The Adaptive Immune System. *NCBI.* [Online] https://www.ncbi.nlm.nih.gov/books/NBK21070/.

497. **Kwon KY, Jo KD, Lee MK, Oh M, Kim EN, Park J, Kim JS, Youn J, Oh E, Kim HT, Oh MY, Jang W.** Low Serum Vitamin D Levels May Contribute to Gastric Dysmotility in de novo Parkinson's Disease. *PubMed.* [Online] Jan 7, 2016. https://www.ncbi.nlm.nih.gov/pubmed/26735311.

498. What causes depression? [Online] http://www.health.harvard.edu/mind-and-mood/what-causes-depression.

499. Vitamin D deficiency linked more closely to diabetes than obesity. *Eurek Alert.* [Online] Feb 23, 2015. https://www.eurekalert.org/pub_releases/2015-02/tes-vdd021815.php.

500. **Bergman, Peter,1 Susanne Sperneder,2 Jonas Höijer,3 Jenny Bergqvist,2,4 and Linda Björkhem-Bergman1,2,*.** Low Vitamin D Levels Are Associated with Higher Opioid Dose in Palliative Cancer Patients – Results from an Observational Study in Sweden. *PLOS ONE.* [Online] 2015. https://www.ncbi.nlm.nih.gov/pmc/articles/PMC4446094/.

501. **Moritz, Andreas.** *Heal yourself with the Sunlight.*

502. **J Brent Richards, Ana M Valdes, Jeffrey P Gardner, Dimitri Paximadas, Masayuki Kimura, Ayrun Nessa, Xiaobin Lu, Gabriela L Surdulescu, Rami Swaminathan, Tim D Spector, and Abraham Aviv.** Higher serum vitamin D concentrations are associated with longer leukocyte telomere length in women2. *PubMed.* [Online] Jan 14, 2008. https://www.ncbi.nlm.nih.gov/pmc/articles/PMC2196219/.

503. **Mohsen Mazidi,corresponding author1,2 Erin D. Michos,3,4 and Maciej Banach5,6.** The association of telomere length and serum 25-hydroxyvitamin D levels in US adults: the National Health and Nutrition Examination Survey. *PubMed.* [Online] Feb 1, 2017. https://www.ncbi.nlm.nih.gov/pmc/articles/PMC5206371/.

504. **Jones, G.** Why dialysis patients need combination therapy with both cholecalciferol and a calcitriol analogs. *PubMed.* [Online] May 2010. https://www.ncbi.nlm.nih.gov/pubmed/20492584.

505. Vitamin D increases the number of blood stem cells during embryonic development. *EurekAlert.* [Online] Oct 2016. https://www.eurekalert.org/pub_releases/2016-10/cp-vdi100316.php.

506. **Cowan, Thomas, MD.** The Heart is Not a Pump. *Chelsea Green Publishing.* [Online] Nov 2016. http://www.chelseagreen.com/blogs/author-thomas-cowan-heart-pump/.

507. **Koskinen, Timo,Tapio Kuoppala, Risto Tuimala.** Amniotic fluid 25-hydroxyvitamin D concentrations in normal and complicated pregnancy. [Online] Jan 1986. http://www.ejog.org/article/0028-2243(86)90039-0/abstract.

508. Newspaper. *http://the-newspapers.com/2016/07/20/in-the-human-brain-discovered-quantum-tunnel.* [Online] July 20, 2016.

509. **van, Ward Paul.** *The Soul Genome.* s.l. : Wheatmark Inc., 2008.

510. The Cosmic Octave. [Online] 2012. http://www.planetware.de/octave/.

511. **Meisner, Gary.** Music and the Fibonacci Sequence and Phi. *Golden Number.* [Online] May 4, 2012. https://www.goldennumber.net/music/.

512. **Watson J.D. and Crick F.H.C. .** double helix. *nature.* [Online] Apr 1953. http://www.nature.com/nature/dna50/archive.html.

513. **Ho, Mae-Wan , M.D.** The Real Bioinformatics Revolution, Proteins and Nucleic Acids Singing to One Another? *Science in Society.* [Online] http://www.i-sis.org.uk/TheRealBioinformaticsRevolution.php Proteins and Nucleic Acids Singing to One Another.

514. **Lindberg, David C.** *Theories of Vision from Al-kindi to Kepler.* s.l. : University of Chicago Press, 1981.

515. [Online] http://www.thehopeandfaithfoundation.org/sacred-meaning-of-the-octagon-.

516. SACRED MEANING OF THE OCTAGON. *The Hope and Faith Foundation.* [Online] 2012. http://www.thehopeandfaithfoundation.org/sacred-meaning-of-the-octagon-.

517. **Mosca, Ralph S.** Potential Uses of Cord Blood in Cardiac Surgery. [Online] 2012. https://www.hindawi.com/journals/jbt/2012/568132/.

518. History of stem cell research. *About Stem Cells.* [Online] 2010. http://stemcell.childrenshospital.org/about-stem-cells/history/.

519. **De Kok IJ1, Hicok KC, Padilla RJ, Young RG, Cooper LF.** Effect of vitamin D pretreatment of human mesenchymal stem cells on ectopic bone formation. *PubMed.* [Online] 2006. https://www.ncbi.nlm.nih.gov/pubmed/16836173.

520. **Murnaghan, Ian BSc (hons), MSc .** Cord Blood Stem Cells. *Explore Stem Cells.* [Online] Oct 29, 2012. http://www.explorestemcells.co.uk/cordbloodstemcells.html.

521. **Ahmed FE1, Setlow RB, Grist E, Setlow N.** DNA damage, photorepair, and survival in fish and human cells exposed to UV radiation. [Online] 1993. https://www.ncbi.nlm.nih.gov/pubmed/8393402.

522. H3O2 Research. *H3O2 Water.* [Online] http://h3o2water.com/research/.

523. **Popp, Dr. Fritz-Albert, Bröckers Matthias.** *Die Botschaft der Nahrung.* s.l. : ZWEITAUSENDEINS Versand- Dienst GmbH, 2005. ISBN-13: 978-3861503194.

524. Human Genome. *Science Daily.* [Online] https://www.sciencedaily.com/terms/human_genome.htm.

525. Narrowband ultraviolet B phototherapy for patients with refractory uraemic pruritus: a randomized controlled trial. *PubMed.* [Online] Sep 2011. https://www.ncbi.nlm.nih.gov/pubmed/21668425.

526. http://www.bluroom.com/. [Online]

527. **Herrmann, Ned.** What is the function of the various brainwaves? *Sceintific American.* [Online] https://www.scientificamerican.com/article/what-is-the-function-of-t-1997-12-22/.

528. The Measurement of Brain Waves. *psych.westminster.edu.* [Online] http://www.psych.westminster.edu/psybio/BN/Labs/Brainwaves.htm.

529. **Beloussov, V.L. Voeikov,V.S. Martynyuk.** *Biophotonics and Coherent Systems in Biology.* s.l. : Springer, 1989 - 2007. ISBN: 13 978-0387-28417-0.

Index

4

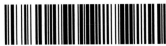

Made in the USA
Lexington, KY
17 October 2017